CUBAN MEDICINE

CUBAN MEDICINE

ROSS DANIELSON

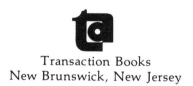

Transaction Books
New Brunswick, New Jersey

Library of Congress Catalog Number: 76-1768
ISBN: 0-87855-114-X (cloth)
Printed in the United States of America

Library of Congress Cataloging in Publication
Data
Danielson, Roswell S.
Cuban medicine.

    Includes bibliographical references and
index.
    1. Medicine—Cuba—History. 2. Social
medicine—Cuba—History. 3. Medical care—
Cuba—History. 4. Medicine, State—Cuba—
History. I. Title. [DNLM: 1. Health services—
History—Cuba. 2. History of medicine—Cuba.
WZ70 DC9 D1c] R475. C9D36 610′ .97291
76-1768 ISBN 0-87855-114-X

Contents

List of Illustrations

Foreword

Eliot Freidson

This book by Ross Danielson is a description of the development of health services in Cuba from the days of the first European colonists to the present. As such, it is a history, but it is not a work in the tradition of the history of medicine. Rather, it is a history of the development of health-related institutions, which include those of the medical profession, but which by no means restricts itself to clinical medicine and its special perspective on illness and its management. Indeed, since his focus is on the substance and organization of health services, and their relationship to the health needs of the entire population of Cuba, much of his discussion dwells on facets of history which have little direct relationship to medical science — the political and economic powers that determine health policy in the nation.

No description is ever neutral; every description is an argument. Every description must be finite and selective in what it includes, and in creating it one also argues, implicitly or explicitly, that what has been chosen for inclusion is more essential, more "true" than what was not included. Danielson's choice is to emphasize health services rather than medical discovery, to evaluate health services, not by the technical sophistication of isolated medical centers, but by the degree to which services are made available to all members of a population, poor as well as rich, rural as well as urban. His emphasis on the development of public health and social medicine creates a rather different picture than would an emphasis on advances in clinical and surgical knowledge and technique. By his choice of what to describe, he implicitly argues that the distribution of available health-related techniques to all who need it is a more critical measure of social progress than is the discovery of knowledge and technique alone.

However, I am sure that neither Danielson nor anyone else would argue for a forced choice. In his history, the development of secularized medical practice and medical education is considered important enough to be called one of the four major medical revolutions of Cuba. So too is the development of scientific hygiene and epidemiology, and the clinical applications of nineteenth century science. The achievement of knowledge and technique is not unimportant; the point is that such achievement has little meaning for humanity at large if it is not for the benefit of all. Distributing or applying knowledge and technique is a different problem from that of discovery. It does concern medical science, but also, wittingly or unwittingly also concerns the use of economic and political power to mobilize and organize the efforts of those who can apply such science. Thus, in Danielson's scheme, what he calls the third and fourth medical revolutions of Cuba were not characterized by signal scientific discoveries, but by changes in the economic and political structure of health-related institutions which were of importance to the way health care could be organized and distributed.

His belief in the importance of bringing health services to all the people leads Danielson to be extremely sympathetic to the revolution of 1959 and the present revolutionary regime, for it has undertaken a vigorous campaign to extend effective health services to the poor and to the rural areas, which had received rather little in times past. Given this sympathy, and his concern less with the comfort of the professions and more with the health of all the people of Cuba, I have no doubt that some portions of his evaluation of the state of health services before the present government will cause disagreement among those of different sympathies. Furthermore, some of what he barely discusses in his exposition—such as the human cost of the reorganization of university and medical school faculties—would no doubt be discussed at length by critics of the present government. This is inevitable, a function of the analytical and ideological elements of choice to be found in any coherent description. His basic values are stated with candor, and so his standpoint or perspective is clear.

Throughout his exposition, there is a rare quality of sympathy and compassion for all the earnest and honest health reformers, physicians, and medical faculty of Cuba, regardless of their political orientation. Above particularistic ideology, Danielson is committed to the cultivation of human potential and to the creation of an environment in which it can flourish. Anything and anyone contributing to this potential is to be admired. Thus, he admires Romay's efforts in the first half of the nineteenth century to advance the use of scientific medicine, even though he was one of the entrenched aristocrats whose position presupposed economic reliance on slavery. He applauds the wiping out of yellow fever, even though it was performed under the auspices of an occupying military force. And he argues that many of the physicians who left Cuba after the revolution were not as venal and selfish as those who remained characterized them. Rather, these refugees were overwhelmed by the too-swift pace of events: he even guesses that, under less stressful circumstances, many could have found a satisfying and productive professional role in their native land under its revolutionary government.

In his way, Danielson has also written a profoundly conservative book, conservative in the sense that he shows the traditional roots of ostensibly untraditional, revolutionary reforms. He shows how circumstances created by a government without commitment to established institutions are nonetheless linked with tradition. He finds the roots of present-day health policies in Cuba in the public health revolution of Carlos Finlay in particular, and in the development of epidemiology and social medicine in general. He shows how and why mutualism—private, prepaid health service mutual aid associations for particular segments of the population—developed, and how it prepared the way for the national reorganization of health care. Indeed, in many ways he seems to see the organization of health services in present-day Cuba as the triumphant culmination of the struggles of many past humane and dedicated Cubans to improve the public health. He sees it as a permanent joining of scientific clinical medicine to social medicine by a social and political framework built into, extending through, and binding together medical schools, hospitals, polyclinics and local community groups to a common purpose. But, unlike conventional conservatives, he implies that such permanent unification of the entire health system would not have occurred without the revolution of 1959.

Danielson's history of health services in Cuba presents us with a study of grand past intentions and, at best, only modest past advances. Romay secularized medical education in Cuba so that it could be open to receive and teach the growing body of new scientific knowledge, but the faculty remained deeply committed to privilege, nepotism, and rigid departmental fiefdoms which resisted the organizational changes necessary to synthesize and adequately teach that new knowledge. Furthermore, while the extraordinary advances of scientific medicine in the late nineteenth and early twentieth centuries were indeed taught to medical students, they employed their knowledge largely for the benefit of the privileged few who lived in Havana and could afford either private or mutual society subscription fees.

Similarly, the possibility for preventing infectious disease, to which Carlos Finlay contributed by his discovery that the mosquito was the carrier of yellow fever, was severely limited. Success in virtually eliminating yellow fever seems to have required the use of the resources, including military force, of a foreign occupying army. When the subsequent national government formed a civilian public health agency, it quickly degenerated into a corrupt civil service which seems to have brought, at best, only nominal benefits to the people. When the anachronistic organization of the work of most Cuban physicians created such great difficulties as to lead to something like a medical trade union which could participate in general strikes, the outcome was not one of benefit to all. Once the federation gained its minimum salary scales, increased employment security, and other benefits, its progressive goals remained stymied by selfish interests. Throughout Cuba's prerevolutionary existence as a nation, its governments were too corrupt, too brutalized or too indebted for their election to a multitude of selfish interests to be able to sustain a vigorous public role in health care. Rationalizing the organization of health services, and bringing a significant volume and range of services into the rural areas occurred only after the revolution of 1959.

Thus, in the face of the history of efforts at the reform and extension of health services found in this book, it would appear that in Cuba, extensive and far-reaching reforms such as Danielson describes could not have taken place with such speed without a revolutionary government primarily indebted to urban and rural workers, rather than to members of the commercial and political establishment. Perhaps they could have taken place over time without revolution, but certainly not as quickly or as comprehensively. Creating a tightly organized, rational national system precludes commitment to established institutions. The very fact that a revolution of the left has no commitment to the maintenance and repair of established institutions, with their crazy-quilt patchwork of arrangements inherited from times past, leaves it able to make some kinds of reforms very quickly.

The acid test of any reform, however, lies in its future, not the legislation establishing it, and neat tables of organization. One must see reform not as noun but as verb, not as birth but as development, not as event but as process. The acid test lies in the way the plan and the organization age. While peaceful reform remains bound up and tied down by established commitments and so cannot make really sweeping changes, revolutionary reform may become transformed in time by conventionalization, its reforms rather more tempered and less sweeping and radical than originally intended. Indeed, by the nature of the case an establishment is eventually created, and vested interests develop within it. The impetus of crisis eventually fades. While initial achievements which transform some of the basic conditions of human life—like those connected with the classic public health diseases and conditions—are likely to be permanent, the character of subsequent achievement may be far more modest. Danielson has shown us how health services in Cuba came to be what they are today. What they will be tomorrow remains to be seen.

CUBAN MEDICINE

1
Introduction

HISTORICAL PERSPECTIVE

Toward the end of my first visit to Cuba in fall 1968, assisted by many interviews and my briefcase weighted by statistics, I became increasingly aware of a gaping hole in my understanding of the Cuban health system and in my ability to describe the system to others, especially to a cynical North American audience. What I had seen during my ten weeks in Cuba had seemed real enough, but the words I had for friends and colleagues back home had the unconvincing sound of new jargon and formulas. I was prepared to describe the Cuban system, but I could not explain it. My description thus had a kind of hollowness, and the "new physician," for example, who went "wherever the revolution called," could easily have been mistaken for a socialist robot. I could gain credibility, I was told, by "toning down my comments." The point, I realized, was that rhetoric, formulas, and new values sounded and looked real in Cuba because they were nestled within a specific historical setting. To communicate that reality I would have to communicate that context, but this was ineffectively communicated by a simple introductory digression on the history of the Cuban Revolution. To speak of the Cuban Revolution as external to the health system, which I had seen as a very dynamic sphere of social activity, turned the evolving health sector into a passive, albeit important, by-product of the political and economic order. Nothing less would suffice than a history of revolution *in* the health sector.

I set myself in the ensuing years to work along two lines of historical research. First, I endeavored to learn about prerevolutionary Cuba by interviewing Cuban physicians who had emigrated to the United States; second,

I embarked on a three-year study of historical documents that could be found in U.S. libraries (notably the New York Academy of Medicine Library). Finally, after most of the present volume was completed, I again had an opportunity to visit Cuba in March 1976, by invitation of the Ministry of Public Health. Unfortunately, all of the materials collected during that two-week visit were confiscated by U.S. Customs, who imposed the condition for their release that I submit to unlimited interrogation concerning my trip. I refused to submit to this blackmail (which continues to this date, February 1978) and I have spent the interim updating my manuscript and fighting unsuccessfully with U.S. Customs. Now, like any researcher, I am forced to leave a number of loose ends and unturned stones. Sadly, many of the loose ends of research are the painful consequences of meager personal resources, absence of institutional support, and of the many impediments which U.S. foreign policy has placed on communications with and travel to Cuba. In spite of such obstacles, enough history has been uncovered so that the story of health system development from early colonial times to the present may be told in a relatively convincing fashion. A well-told story is admittedly not a high level of historical or sociological explanation, but it is a beginning which is markedly superior to an ahistorical analysis of contemporary structures.

It is only through analysis of historical process that one can begin to comprehend such important matters in Cuba as the legacy of institutional concentration in Havana, the cultural reasons for not developing feldshers in the socialist period, the social bases for conflict and compromise within the medical profession, or the process by which conflict itself has formed the contemporary consciousness and ideology of Cuban health workers. Without an understanding of such matters, it is hardly possible to say what the revolution has actually been; for revolution is not outcome, but process; not statistics, but work and struggle. This work and struggle cannot be explained merely by faraway goals and political hues, but by an examination of the confrontation between real people, armed with ideas and politics, and the concrete problems that are thrust upon them by history.

If historical perspective is as important as I contend it is, it is somewhat enigmatic, that in this, the twentieth year of the Cuban Revolution, historical perspective has found so little substantive expression in the literature on health promotion in Cuba. To my knowledge, the best overall view of the structure and process of health services, with a perspective on sociopolitical context, is still a 1972 article by Vicente Navarro.[1] Excepting certain work by Cuban medical historians, the most substantive treatment of a particular line of historical events within the health system is Willis Butler's 1974 article on medical education in Cuba.[2] In-house accounts by the Cuban Ministry of Public Health (MINSAP), largely unavailable to the North American reader, include valuable historical observations, statistical trends, and the like, but historical analysis is usually quite secondary to an immediate descriptive objective. This is not true of a substantial amount of work in medical history that has been supported by the Scientific Council of MINSAP, but here the perspectives have been highly specialized, most of them centered on biographical objectives, some of them focused on specific institutions and periods, and almost always concerned with early prerevolutionary days. Meanwhile, the impressive attempts at comprehensive analysis of general Cuban history, which include a variety of health-related data and trends, have tended to treat health data as if they were wholly disconnected from a line of important institutional development and dynamic health policy. Statistics are analyzed as products or "measures" of the revolution. Although this evaluation has been broadly favorable, the work of health promotion has, nonetheless, remained barely visible to the outside observer — an inattention which does not correspond to the importance which is commonly attributed by the people of Cuba or budgeted by the revolutionary government.

Setting aside a discussion of the forces which influence the research efforts of North American colleagues, perhaps the most important reason for the absence of the kind of historical analysis that I have in mind is that those who have the best view of the whole process — the Cuban health activists themselves — are simply too busy doing other, more important things. Moreover, their motivation would, in any case, probably be somewhat different from my own, precisely because through experience Cuban reality already makes sense to them. From such a view, the task of history will tend to be perceived as the chronicling or recording of events, rather than the somewhat different objective of trying to make sense out of reality by delving in social and historical analysis.

INTERVIEWS AND DIRECT OBSERVATION

My discussion of contemporary Cuba is based primarily on direct observation of the Cuban health system and extensive, unstructured interviews during ten weeks in fall 1968 and two weeks of spring 1976 in several areas of Cuba and at various levels and subunits of the Ministry of Public Health. Additionally, in summer 1969 and, less systematically, in the years following, I conducted interviews with Cuban physicians who had emigrated to the United States. Several of the emigrant physicians had occupied high medical and public health positions in the prerevolutionary years; others came from rather humble medical careers. Some had very recently arrived in the United States.[3]

Those whom I interviewed — revolutionaries and emigrant physicians — were gracious, open, and generally self-critical. I found myself deeply moved by the Cubans who are busy mixing great amounts of hard work, imagination, and revolutionary enthusiasm. Hardly less compassion, however, did I feel for the Cubans who, for whatever reasons, have left their homeland. The marginal situation of many Cuban physicians in the United States is perhaps no more comfortable than different conditions of marginality which may have been experienced in rapidly changing Cuba. I found the emigrant physicians to be, like their counterparts, good, humanely motivated people, people I came to care for and respect. The difference between emigrant physicians and those in Cuba was less a difference between good people and bad people as it was a difference between people of two moral worlds. The new moral world belongs to the people in Cuba: the old moral world belongs, in a sense, to the emigrants. An important aim of this work is to understand those two worlds and thus the meaning of the revolution which is driving them apart.

Interviews with emigrant physicians supplemented weaknesses in the impressions I obtained in Cuba, especially with regard to the prerevolutionary years and the initial period of transition. By 1968, after ten years of revolution, so much had changed, so much had happened, that in Cuba the prerevolutionary years already appeared more remote and hazy than a mere ten years might suggest. By 1968, and certainly by 1976, many of the new Cuban physicians were young people whose major formation had been within the revolution. Today this category includes three-fourths of all physicians. Thus for many Cubans the prerevolutionary years already appeared as the Dark Ages. The opposite tendency existed among many emigrants: the prerevolutionary years were either the "good old days" or otherwise years of promise and intrinsic value. More important, there were those, on both sides of the Florida Straits, who were honestly and evenly critical and praising of both past and present.

In light of the differences between the two groups of physicians interviewed, it is of considerable methodological significance that I uncovered little disagreement over questions of fact. Disagreement centered on questions of interpretation and on conflicting values and interests.

It is important, in sharing my judgments based upon interviews and travel in Cuba, to identify the role that I projected, or thought I projected, as an interviewer. It is also appropriate that I make explicit certain values that I hold as well as what I believe to be their methodological significance.

In 1968, when I traveled to Cuba as a member of Students for a Democratic Society, my guides from the Cuban Friendship Institute introduced me everywhere as a young revolutionary. This no doubt colored my interviews, tending to make them highly informal and leading my interviewees to ask me as many questions as I asked them. On my return visit in 1976, I was treated differently, owing to an invitation from the Ministry of Public Health that was based on my academic credentials. The man who came to pick me up at the airport on that occasion exclaimed, when I ventured to introduce myself, "Oh, I was expecting an old man with a grey beard!" In 1976, then, my interviews tended to be more formal. This reflected the different identity which I then projected and also the highly focused and efficient schedule of the second visit. In the meanwhile, my political views had matured more than they had changed: I sympathize with the broad objectives of the Cuban Revolution, and I am actively committed to the socialist movement in my own country. Whatever the complications of such a role, I am personally convinced that my politics support, and are supported by, a scientific orientation toward argument and evidence.

I reject the naive view of value-free sociology, so predominant when I was a student, which urges one not to be partisan while being a sociologist and which pressures one to dishonestly write the final report in the value-free style, suppressing any information about one's inelegant involvement with the subject under study. Science is not an individualistic enterprise dependent upon the objectivity of individuals; science is rather a collective enterprise dependent upon objectivity as a social process, the process by which opinions of different people tend to converge under the weight of evidence. This study is not to be entitled "The TRUTH about Health Care in Cuba;" it is only part of a process of people trying to understand that reality. I will aid this process by striving to be honest and clear.

This is not to deny that taking a politically committed role, or any other role, has many implications for the production of knowledge and judgements. One is led to ask certain questions rather than others and to focus on certain aspects of reality. A given role, moreover, makes it possible to observe and experience in ways that otherwise would be difficult or impossible. And involvement, with all its well-known pitfalls, helps one to care enough to look carefully.

In August 1968, I traveled to Cuba as a member of a 37-person rank and file delegation of Students for a Democratic Society. For the first two weeks I participated in the collective activities of that delegation. In the remaining eight weeks, with the assistance of the Cuban Institute of Friendship and the Ministry of Public Health, I organized many interviews and visits to institutions, and I sometimes made visits without prior arrangement or official sanction. In any case, I was almost always introduced with reference to political credentials, which in an intensely political society invariably served to break the ice. It helped of course that I spoke Spanish, and many hours were spent in casual discussion with students, friends, workers, medical personnel, and members of various revolutionary organizations.

My identification as a former member of an SDS delegation to Cuba and my favorable impressions of contemporary Cuba must have distressed some of my emigrant hosts when I turned to them in 1969. But this irritation was outweighed by their favorable impression of my obvious interest in learning from their point of view. Moreover, by 1969, most of the emigrant physicians had come to recognize many good, if not for them redeeming, qualities of the revolution. Most were eager to find out what I had seen in Cuba, and I was surprised to learn that the émigrés knew very little about the evolving structure and activities of health promotion in Cuba. Many, for example, thought that mutualist medical programs (prepaid plans, important to many Cubans in prerevolutionary Havana) had been ended in 1961. In fact, mutualist programs were still in existence, albeit greatly reformed, in 1968. By contrast, in Cuba I had acquired hardly any idea of the influential and complex role of mutualist organization either before or after 1959. My interviews with émigré physicians were valuable in lending insight to the period of early revolutionary transition and the personal meaning of certain prerevolutionary institutions, struggles, and traditions. I identified a glimmering sentiment among older physicians of personal connection to a medical history that predates even the republican era in Cuba.

Upon my second arrival to Cuba, my immediate host, Dr. Francisco Rojas Ochoa (head of the statistical section of the Ministry of Public Health) reviewed my research objectives and helped me organize an intensive schedule of interviews with more than forty persons. He also organized visits to numerous institutions in Havana and Matanzas provinces. Focusing primarily on changes in the community health center (area polyclinic) and on the new local organs of Cuban government (assemblies of people's power), I was able to witness recent transformations in the organization of health care and society which have sprung from the social dynamics that were in motion in 1968. The visit enabled me to confirm certain conclusions that had been based entirely on émigré perspectives; I found a unique opportunity to learn about the recent history of dentistry in Cuba. Review of documents at the Museum of the History of Science and interviews with older medical activists served to verify tenuous conclusions and correct certain errors of the early manuscript, particularly one of omission: *I had earlier failed to note the exclusion or segregation of blacks in most of the prepaid medical plans of prerevolutionary Cuba.* In sum, the second visit allowed revisions and expansion of the previous manuscript, as well as the addition of the section which treats the contemporary period (after 1971) of "medicine in the community."

HISTORICAL DOCUMENTS

Personal interviews often raised as many new questions as they answered and thus in 1969, when I discovered a great store of available historical documents in the library of the New York Academy of Medicine, I became hopelessly committed to an even larger project of uncovering the past.

It seemed impossible, for a long time, to ever prepare myself to write the historical sections until, finally, I gathered together a small store of key sources and notes and went off to write a first draft. Thus I lean heavily on a few key sources, somewhat moderated by later revisions. Unfortunately, many important sources have been unavailable by means of interlibrary loan. Hugh Thomas's prodigious history of Cuba was an indispensble aid, a brilliantly analyzed (although not infallible) source and guide to data on Cuban history.[4] In Havana, the venerable medical historian César Rodríguez Expósito, after an impressive tour and interview in the library of the Museum of Medical History, formerly the Cuban Academy of Sciences, gave me several key texts: the complete works of Carlos J. Finlay,[5] the complete works of Tomás Romay,[6] a detailed account of the history of hospitals in Cuba before 1900,[7] a tediously detailed chronology of dentistry,[8] a biography of Joaquín Albarrán,[9] along with Rodríguez Expósito's own account of the establishment of the first ministry of health in Cuba[10] and his biography of Dr. Juan Guiteras.[11] Still another key book was mailed to me after my 1976 visit — the witty, colorful, and informative autobiography of Dr. Mario E. Dihigo.[12] The original sources and biographies brought to life what for me were otherwise coldly remote years and helped me to respect the struggles and personal efforts that built the Cuban health system.

CONCEPTS OF HEALTH ORGANIZATION

The purpose here is not to provide an exhaustive list of definitions for technical terms, but rather to set forth the bare ingredients of a sociological perspective which has been in the back of my mind in the course of my study and analysis. It may or may not be helpful for the reader to share such a perspective but it is offered in the hope that it may contribute to the perception of whole systems in process, which on an abstract level is what this book is about. In the remainder of the work, however, I have tried to use concrete rather than technical language. I have intended that the more abstract forays into sociological analysis be given in sections that are independent of the substantive discussion. *The reader may elect to skim or skip this section entirely, without significantly jeopardizing substantive communication.*

Health Organizations and the Health System

The health system of a society may usefully be thought of as the collection of all health organizations in that society and their interrelations. By health organization is meant any organization (or suborganization) which has as its primary, defining, and justifying goal the positive transformation of directly health-related aspects of people and their environment. Hospitals, medical schools, dental clinics, and sanitation departments are examples. The health system then is the largest (conceptually) possible health organization, of which all other health organizations are parts.

Diagram 1.1
A Health Organization and Its Environment

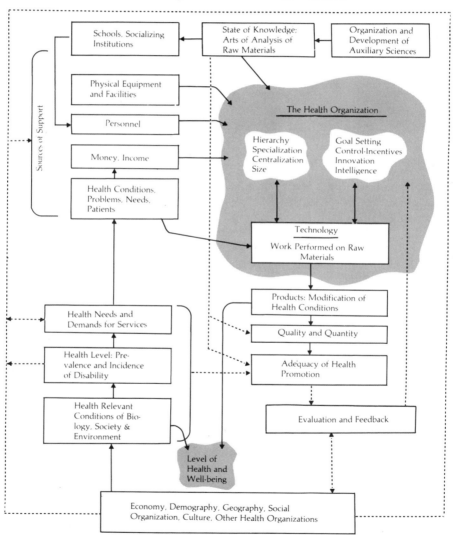

Health organizations may be seen to differ in many respects, some of which are indicated or suggested in the diagrams which follow. Diagram 1 focuses our attention on the input-output context of health organizations. Using the factory analogy, organizations may first be characterized by the raw material inputs, the transformation of which constitutes the identifying work of the organization. Some health organizations perform work on patients; other health organizations work on other health-relevant conditions, such as sanitation or health education. Choosing another simplifying definition, how the work is done constitutes the technology of the organization. The technology implies supportive inputs to the organization such as money or other forms of budgetary power, personnel, facilities, and supplies. A variable process of evaluation, both internal and external to the organization, may be thought to have two output components — evaluations of quality and adequacy. The quality of the work done is evaluated by comparison with idealized standards derived from what is known about the health problems which constitute the raw material inputs. The adequacy of health promotion work is evaluated with respect to three factors: the quality of individual services, their relation to the health needs of the area-constituency served, and the resource limitations imposed by scarcity and unequal priorities. Quality then, is a kind of idealized concept while adequacy is the associated pragmatic concept. Or, simply, adequacy is quality modified by pragmatism. The ability of the organization to deliver adequate services will depend not only upon the internal structure of the organization, but also upon the external structure of the organization, upon the quality and adequacy of the organizations which supply the supportive inputs — medical schools, training programs, drug and equipment manufacturers — and the ability of health organization to successfully demand supportive inputs. Supportive institutions, in turn, depend upon, and are part of, the overall status of economy, culture, and politics of the society itself. Quality and adequacy of health promotion work will be evaluated by the people served, by those who do the work, by other health organizations, and by influential publics. The effect of various assessments of adequacy depends upon the existence of real feedback mechanisms, the interdependence of relevant parts, the distribution of power, and the generation of social movements.

The focus on health and well-being in Diagram 1.1 is intended to emphasize that the health system includes only part of the health-relevant aspects of a society. Therefore, rational resource allocation for health promotion sets limits for the health system in accord with a range of social priorities. Diagram 1.2 suggests a system of interrelatedness, for example, between public health and commodity production, where both contribute to the health level and to each other. Production and health level provide inputs to other social subsystems, such as education, politics, and social stratification. These systems similarly provide significant inputs to the health system, to production, and to one another. These inputs, however, may be positive or negative, or the positive or negative consequence may depend on a combination of inputs. For example, industrialization led first to slums and deteriorating health conditions until sanitary measures, improved distribution of food, and other social developments, not unrelated to industrialization, made possible an improved relation between production and health. The point is that, whatever the specific substance of interrelatedness, there does exist a system of phenomena that relates to health, to health organizations, and to the health system. Health promotion by a society is not limited to direct investments in the health system, and alternative investments for health promotion, when consciously identified, offer wide degrees of debate in virtually every society. In a sense, when the idealized health planner looks at society, the whole of society becomes the health system. But the dizzying height of this perspective probably helps insure the widespread inattention to such a broad view of health promotion; at best its approximation is implicit in the actions of some political activists and social reformers. In Cuba, the social perspective of health promotion is approximated in the goals of socialist planning, and in the ideological work of political cadre who seek to prevent the ascendency of narrow interest group or technocratic perspectives. The broad view is explicitly assumed when the health planning of the Ministry of Public Health is evaluated by the Central Planning Board, Cuba's highest planning body. Someday, perhaps, a role will emerge for a new kind of epidemiologist whose perspective will be incorporated into the process of social planning.

Diagram 1.2
Input-Output Relations between Production and Public Health

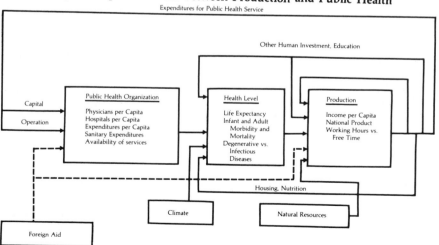

The drawing of lines and arrows in our diagrams is partially arbitrary. Health organizations, like all social systems, involve two-way, direct and indirect relationships among the various parts and variables. Here the directional lines indicate the flow of interaction which interests me. Nothing is meant to imply harmony or continuity among the parts. The flow of arrows in Diagram 1.1 indicates the flow from what I consider to be the generally more deterministic aspects of the system to the less deterministic aspects. Given the limits set by the "hard" variables of demography and economics, the more precise state of the system and its probable future are given by the "soft" variables of social structure, political composition, and culture. Change may be initiated in any part of a health organization, from within or from without, but each bit of change can go only so far until it meets with appropriate responses from other parts of the system. Thus each position in the system is also a potential source of rigidity and reaction. Depending on the context, the nature of change initiated, and the point of origin in the system, the initiation of change may be smoothly effected, effected after great conflict and tension, unresolved with chronic antagonism, or smoothly suppressed. The probability distribution of such outcomes among the parts of an organization and its environment is essentially the distribution of power or influence. Sometimes the power to veto is distributed such that little significant change may be initiated anywhere, and, mysteriously, the "powerful"' are often powerless. This was a prevailing characteristic, as will be seen, in prerevolutionary Cuba.

Permanent Tension for Change

However, in health organizations we may assume change in the factors of adequacy: (1) the state of the applied arts of analysis of health conditions (the basis for quality determination), (2) health conditions and health needs, and (3) the reasonable availability of resources to be allocated to the support of health promotion. Consequently the health system exists under conditions of permanent tension for change.

The Marxist general theory of social change provides an appropriate model for such systems of internal tension, and it is therefore helpful to have in mind a correspondence between the categories of a Marxist model and those of any pragmatic model used for social analysis. Here, for instance, the factors of adequacy defined in the paragraph above, are precisely the forces of production in what I would consider to be a Marxist model[13] of the health organization (see Diagram 1.3). The forces of production — primary, irresistable, initiators of social change — are at once oppressed and liberated by the relations of production (the social structure, roughly speaking) and the ideological superstructure (prevailing social values).

Diagram 1.3
A Marxist Model of Health Promotion System

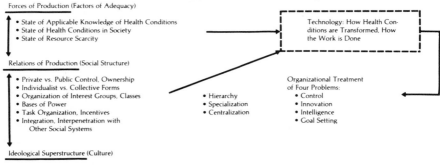

Forces of Production (Factors of Adequacy)

- State of Applicable Knowledge of Health Conditions
- State of Health Conditions in Society
- State of Resource Scarcity

Technology: How Health Conditions are Transformed, How the Work is Done

Relations of Production (Social Structure)

- Private vs. Public Control, Ownership
- Individualist vs. Collective Forms
- Organization of Interest Groups, Classes
- Bases of Power
- Task Organization, Incentives
- Integration, Interpenetration with Other Social Systems

- Hierarchy
- Specialization
- Centralization

Organizational Treatment of Four Problems:
- Control
- Innovation
- Intelligence
- Goal Setting

Ideological Superstructure (Culture)

- Concepts of Health Promotion: Commodity, Privilege, or Human Right; Preventive vs. Curative Focus

- Sense of Purpose or Mission: Charity, Quality Care, Comprehensive Health Care, Positive Health

- Predominant Values of Society and Key Institutions; Egalitarianism vs. Elitism; Collectivism vs. Individualism

In agreement with predictions from the Marxist model, when significant change occurs in the health sector, one or more of the three components of adequacy has either changed or been reinterpreted. Even where change is initiated, say, for reasons of petty power struggle and narrow self interest, the justification usually rests upon consideration of adequacy. That is, the assessment of adequacy is a social process, a product in part of both the relations of production and the ideological superstructure. Thus, a negative assessment of adequacy is historically relevant only insofar as it is accepted by nonapathetic centers of power or gives rise to a social movement for improvement. Depending on the system of social stratification, the process, pressured by the forces of production (or factors of adequacy), is manifest in some form of social conflict.

Technology

The bridge between the forces of production and the relations of production is technology. The complexity of technology depends on the practical homogeneity of the inputs (Are all the patients victims of tuberculosis? Is the iron ore of uniform composition?), and the ease with which the inputs may be analyzed and understood (What do we know about tuberculosis and iron ore?). The ease of analysis depends on the state of the art of analyzing the raw materials, a product of scientific development and applied research. The extremely important determination and definition of the raw material inputs, their volume and homogeneity, are often the product of forces outside the organization, the prevailing social values and needs of key institutions and groups which depend on the work of the health sector. Diagrams 1.4 and 1.5, borrowed and modified from work by

Charles Perrow,[14] usefully categorize technologies according to a theory of interplay of input homogeneity and arts of analysis.

Diagram 1.4
Technology as the Relation between Raw Materials and Analytical Arts

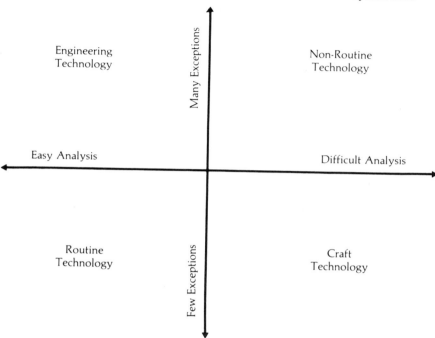

The choice of technology is conditioned by pragmatic and prosaic restraints: changes in the nature of the health conditions treated, the volume of needs or demands for services, external bureaucratic directives, scarcity of resources, and cultural values. Traditionalism or monopoly by a closed profession may inhibit change. Hence, theoretically ideal technologies are not often implemented. The treatment of the mentally ill, a little understood phenomenon, with many exceptional cases, demands such a nonroutine technology (individualized, humane psychotherapy) as to be impractical due to scarcity of resources relative to input volume. The psychiatric institution settles for humane, custodial care, or, worse, brutal custodialism. Problem children in the schools are optimally served by non-routine teaching methods. However, in large classes, the teacher opts either for isolation of problem children or for more repressive means of maintaining routinized instruction. The overworked clinician in the out-patient department of a prestigious hospital settles (wrongly, perhaps) for routinely administered wide-spectrum antibiotics rather than for individualized analysis of each infection. The impoverished nation may reluctantly but wisely settle for non-physicians as primary providers of care. Everywhere organizations operate with less than ideal technology, sometimes less than "quality" but sometimes more than "adequate". And it is here, in the existing technology, that the forces of production and the relations of production meet in a conflict moderated by the prevailing social consciousness, analysis, reform, and revolution.

Diagram 1.5
Technology and Organizational Environment

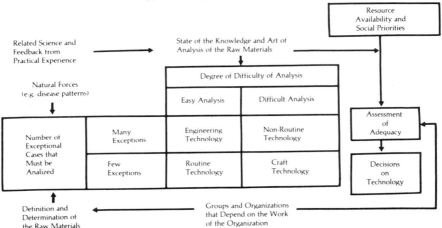

My rather simplified introduction to complex matters should not imply that developments in the understanding of raw materials necessarily move nonroutine technologies toward the routine. Neither does technological change result unambiguously in more adequate health care. Scientific discovery reveals exceptional cases and heterogeneity where none was previously known to exist. While some matters are routinized or moved toward craft and engineering technologies, other areas are created which imply nonroutine technologies. Craft technology may create problems stemming from horizontal specialization. Routinization and engineering technologies compound difficulties arising from multiple hierarchies of personnel of varied skill, training, and incentive level. Engineering technology favors depersonalization. All of the aforementioned processes, accompanied by growing size and volume inputs, enhance the growth of large, complex organizations that are burdened by every conceivable organizational pathology. While quality care is theoretically more available, health care also becomes intimidating, remote, and inaccessible. Every new division of labor, vertical or horizontal, is a potential base for a new interest group. When, as in the case of professional groups, interest groups are interorganizationally and extraorganizationally organized, when health organizations are linked to government and to other powerful institutions, when extensive interdependence develops among health organizations, and when variable patterns of ownership and entrepreneurship are mixed together, the very complex social structures of health systems emerge.

Structural Technology

A very important and complementary alternate approach to such matters follows. While social structure is built upon technology, it is also true that, in a sense, the social structure *is* the technology insofar as it answers the question, how is the work done? Thus the structure itself raises questions of quality and adequacy. The adequacy of the organization of health promotion is determined, in large part, by the state of four permanent problems which beset any complex organization and its parts: goal setting (the sense of mission, integration of different internal goals and operationalization of goals), control (coordination, incentives, work group organization, leadership, and democracy), innovation (potential for individual and collective creativity and for change in purpose and structure), and intelligence ("gathering, processing, interpreting, and communicating the technical and political information needed in the decision making process").[15] An interest of my original research was to understand how such problems are treated by health organizations in Cuba and how the context of the Revolution modifies the effects of specialization, hierarchy, and centralization in the pursuit of a unified health promotion system.

MEDICAL REVOLUTION AND SOCIAL HISTORY

The contemporary Cuban Revolution is neither the first period of social revolution in Cuba nor the first period of fundamental change in the health system. In the following sections, I will discuss three earlier medical revolutions and say something about the respective prerevolutionary periods. The first medical revolution, in the years closing the eighteenth and opening the nineteenth century, juxtaposed scientific method and clinical empiricism against traditional speculative scholasticism. Smallpox vaccination, systematic quarantine, and the beginning of rational public sanitation were introduced. The second medical revolution, at the turn of the next century, effected the eradication of yellow fever and malaria and introduced comprehensive sanitation codes, dramatic advances in the effectiveness of surgery and clinical medicine, and the growth of prepaid clinic and hospital plans of Spanish immigrants. Professional entrenchment was the central thrust of the third medical revolution, consolidated in the years from 1930 to 1945. Professional federations, employment securities, government recognition of professional autonomy, the hegemony of physicians in both private and cooperative prepayment clinics, and the legislation of several social security programs with health care benefits were established. The third revolutionary period was also characterized by growing size, complexity, and capitalization of the health care enterprise, tendencies which foreshadowed the rationalizing organizational thrust of the contemporary period.

Somewhat anticipating my analysis, it is not mere coincidence that each of the three medical revolutions occurred at times of great social upheaval: the curious ascendance of the Cuban bourgeoisie, the ambivalent capture of national independence, and the truncated popular uprising against the Machado dictatorship. The adjectives — curious, ambivalent, and truncated — underscore the impression of incompleteness that one gets from a reading of Cuban history.

Some students of revolution may object to my use of the term "medical revolution" in the periods prior to 1959. By revolution I mean important and radical change;[16] and by offering to identify these revolutions by periods of time, I am using dates to identify change that was highlighted in one or another period. Although not necessarily restricted as a process to specific beginning and end points, one is given opportunity to evaluate whether in fact, an important and radical difference exists between end points of a given period. Of course, by identifying and focusing on revolutionary periods, one may warp the real contours of history. For one is teased toward an implicit understatement of the importance or degree of changes between revolutions. This assertion is not here assumed and the risk of warping history will be lessened by attention, however inadequate, to prerevolutionary and postrevolutionary periods.

Another disclaimer is perhaps appropriate. I have attempted to write a social history, yet a really complete approach of this kind has turned out to be unwieldy, rendering the work less readable and, in any case, introducing too many redundancies with the work of historians who are far more qualified than I to discuss the broad socioeconomic developments of each period. Thus I have settled on a compromise which has its own pitfalls. In each revolutionary period, I have chosen to give sociobiographical attention to the work of outstanding medical figures. This approach introduces the reader to information and analysis that is elsewhere unavailable. In the first medical revolution, from 1790 to 1830, I analyze the role of Tomás Romay; in the second medical revolution, from 1880 to 1910, I analyze the role of Carlos J. Finlay; and in the third medical revolution, from 1925 to 1945, I analyze the Cuban Medical Federation. In the contemporary revolutionary period, I do not use a biographical approach, although more attention to information of this kind would have been neither inappropriate nor uninteresting.

A biographical approach helps, unfortunately, to twist social history into a succession of feats by great men. Similarly, the weak historian's dependence on easily available data favors, as in this work, inordinate attention to the higher social strata of medical practitioners. For the greater part, however, my observations are derived from the writings of each man and not from the analyses of other biographers. In the case of the Cuban Medical Federation, I lean heavily on a detailed account written by an activist of those years.

Finally, let me protest that this is not a study of health and illness but a study of the organization of health promotion. While the former is clearly relevant to the latter, my focus will have the consequence of caring less for attempts at biostatistical precision than for trying to understand how the existence and perception of disability and health system adequacy generate changes in the enterprise of health promotion itself.

ACKNOWLEDGEMENTS

Part of being clear (which usually helps one's honesty) — and an aspect of methodology which is difficult to specify — is becoming acquainted with a broad range of phenomena and developing conceptual tools which are relevant to the subject under study. Such matters may be treated partially in the fashion of acknowledgements. I am particularly indebted to the faculty and fellow graduate students who integrated me into the medical sociology program at the University of Pittsburgh from 1966 to 1969. I am indebted to the conceptually clear and substantively rich analyses of Latin American health systems by Milton Roemer,[17] and of Eastern European health systems by E. Richard Weinerman.[18] Very important to me in developing concepts and theoretical frameworks are certain ideas developed by Charles Perrow and Eliot Freidson. Since 1968, my understanding of the contemporary Cuban system has benefited from the observations of others who have studied health organization there, notably Sally Gattmacher and Vicente Navarro. Russell Morgan, Jr. provided me with bibliography, articles, and documents that he and others gathered in a survey of available information on health care in contemporary Cuba.

No less important among the real world aspects of methodology are one's work incentives. In that sense, this work is also a product of the personal support given to me by Morris Berkowitz, Ray Elling, and José Moreno who convinced me of the merit of relating political and sociological interests. Only Ed Suchman's students can understand what I owe him. Ed Suchman set an unattainable example of workmanship; constructive, insightful criticism; and personal understanding. Still, the strongest motivational support for my work is the attention, trust, and confidence of the Cubans and comrades in Students for a Democratic Society who supported my first trip to Cuba and the personnel of the Cuban Ministry of Public Health who hosted my return visit in 1976. It seems most ambitious to hope that my work can justify the consideration given me by the many persons interviewed.

Without institutional aid of any kind, a ten-year project inevitably posed difficulties for my wife, children, and coworkers. To them I am grateful for their patience and support. Susan Danielson generously assisted in proofreading and gave valuable editorial advice.

NOTES

1. Vicente Navarro, "Health, Health Services, and Health Planning in Cuba," *International Journal of Health Services* 2 (August 1972): 397-432.

2. Willis Butler, "The Undergraduate Education of Physicians in Cuba," *Journal of Medical Education* 48 (September 1973): 846-58.

3. Two physicians expressed a desire that their views remain anonymous. I have therefore eliminated names of *all* persons interviewed. This is not a serious omission, in that most of my argument and discussion is substantiated by a variety of data. Interviews pointed to certain conclusions; but the conclusions do not rest on the interview alone. Interviews were more important in pointing to conclusions than in substantiating them.

4. Hugh Thomas, *Cuba: The Pursuit of Freedom* (New York: Harper and Row, 1971).

5. Carlos J. Finlay, *Obras completas* 3 vols., compiled with a biographical essay by César Rodríquez Expósito, (Havana: Museo Histórico de Ciencias Médicas "Carlos J. Finlay," 1965-1967).

6. Tomás Romay y Chacón, *Obras completas* 2 vols., compiled with an introduction by José López Sánchez, (Havana: Museo Histórico de las Ciencias Médicas "Carlos J. Finlay," 1965).

7. Mario del Pino y de la Vega, "Apuntes para la historia de los hospitales de Cuba (1523 a 1899)," *Cuadernos de Historia de Salud Pública, no. 24*, (Havana: Ministerio de Salud Pública, 1963).

8. José Antonio Martinez-Fortún y Foyo, "Apuntes para la historia de la odontología en Cuba," *Cuadernos de Historia de Salud Pública, no. 23*, (Havana: Ministerio de Salud Pública, 1963).

9. J. Paulís Pagés and M.Y. Monteros-Valdivieso, *Joaquín Albarrán: General artifice de la Urología*, (Havana: Museo Histórico de las Ciencias Médicas "Carlos J. Finlay," 1963).

10. César Rodriguez Expósito, "La primera secretaria de sanidad del mundo se creó en Cuba" *Cuadernos de Historia de Salud Pública, no. 25*, (Havana: Ministerio de Salud Pública, 1964).

11. César Rodriguez Expósito, Dr. *Juan Guiteras* (Havana: Editorial Cubanicán, 1974).

12. Mario E. Dihigo, "Recuerdos de una larga vida," *Cuadernos de Historia de la Salud Pública, no. 60*, (Havana: Ministerio de Salud Pública, 1974). Dihigo graduated from medical school in 1917, practiced briefly in the "El Carreño" sugar mill and in Havana and Bejucal. After 1918, he worked in various settings in Matanzas until his retirement in the mid-1960s.

13. By model, I mean a theory or conceptual framework that exists with respect to some other theory or framework that is analogous in understandable respects to the first. Thus I am not directly applying Marxian theory, which has as its primary focus the whole of society, but rather by analogy I am creating (or at least alluding to) a "Marxian" theory of change in the health sector. It is the latter theory which I am, strictly speaking, applying.

14. Charles Perrow, "A Framework for the Comparative Analysis of Organizations," *American Sociological Review* 32 (April 1967) 2: 194-208; "Hospitals: Technology, Structure, and Goals," in James March (ed.), *Handbook of Organizations* (Chicago: Rand McNally, 1965), 910-71; and "Goals and Power Structures: A Historical Case Analysis," in Eliot Friedson ed., *The Hospital in Modern Society* (New York: The Free Press, 1963), 112-46.

15. Harold Wilensky, *Organizational Intelligence* (New York: Basic Books, 1969), ch. 1.

16. The literature on revolution sometimes falls into the easy error of including a favorite theory in the definition of the word itself (and thus makes impossible the testing of the theory). For my purpose, a minimal definition seems most useful.

17. Milton Roemer, *Medical Care in Latin America* (Washington, D.C.: General Secretariat, Organization of American States, 1963); and "Medical Care and Social Class in Latin America," *Milbank Memorial Fund Quarterly* 42 (July 1964) 3, part I: 54-64.

18. E. Richard Weinerman, M.D., with the assistance of Shirley B. Weinerman, *Social Medicine in Eastern Europe: The Organization of Health Services and the Education of Medical Personnel in Czechoslavakia, Hungary, and Poland*, (Cambridge, Massachusetts: Harvard University Press, 1969).

2
The First Prerevolutionary Period, 1521-1790

EARLY PRACTITIONERS

The early health system in Cuba was a frail transplant of the Spanish system. Its parts were simple and few. The formal or official occupational categories were barber, bleeder, dentist, surgeon, pharmacist, and physician. (Infrequent reference was also made to midwives, bonesetters, and herniotomists.) The jealously disputed working boundaries of the early professions were legally unclear and often circumstantially irrelevant. The barber, on the bottom of the presumed hierarchy of skills, sometimes bled his clients, extracted their teeth, and performed an infrequent postmortem caesarian section.[1] It is no wonder, therefore, that the barber also prescribed or concocted medicines for his patients when they became really sick. The dentist (tooth-puller or *sacamuelas*) as a separate specialist hardly existed in Cuba before 1800 because he was so frequently intruded upon by the surgeon.[2] Pulling teeth was probably in fact the surgeon's most effective operation, followed by, one must generously suppose, the setting of fractures. The trappings of the physician were more likely to include one or two classical medical treatises, some knowledge of Latin, and a formal scholastic education rather than simple apprenticeship. Formal education, of course, suggested the economic means and social status which made education accessible. But while the physician was more erudite and possessed an unintelligible scholastic jargon and disease typology, it should not be imagined that he offered more productive resources of cure.

Speculative medical scholasticism was the medicine of Cuba's sixteenth, seventeenth, and eighteenth century physicians — a galenic metaphysics of vital fluids, bleeding techniques, balsams, and purgatives.

21

That the curative powers of Spanish practitioners were not significantly greater than those of the native Siboney and African folk healers is suggested, although hardly proven, by an inventory of a physician's storeroom, circa 1515.

Next to the learned texts of Galen, Nicandrus, and Hippocrates were the following ingredients: "boiled barley juice, Arabic concoctions of ten, twenty, and more ingredients; coral, pearl, and hyacinth confections; powdered snake meat and snake oil; toad dust; spider oil; and the excrement and urine of different animals."[3]

The Spanish medical circumstance was not unique in Europe. A century later, in 1618, the first London Pharmacopea offered, from among a compendium of some two thousand items, the following nutritious remedies: "snake meat pills, dried fox lungs for respiration problems, bear grease to make hair grow, snake oil to loosen muscles, material scraped from the brain of a convict who had died in chains, crab eyes, human sweat, spider web, and oil of newborn puppies boiled with bits of earth."[4]

Improvisers

The not so lamentable early shortage of physicians in Cuba left wide room for other legal practitioners, especially barbers and surgeons, and many extralegal or informally trained practitioners - pretenders or improvisers of every kind, as well as friars and folk practitioners. Sometimes more and sometimes less dangerous than the physician, their services were at least available in the early Cuban period. The prestige, in fact, of folk practitioners sometimes rivaled that of the physician. Early explorers were so impressed by native herb healers that they were often the preferred source of medical assistance. Cortés, it is reported, held the native healers in such high esteem that he begged the king not to send physicians.[5] Later, the widespread prestige of native healers and their enjoyment of religious authority among their own people caused an alarmed Church to forbid their practice. But in Cuba, considering the early and severe decimation of her native population by conquest, forced labor, and epidemic, the initial influence of native practitioners was probably out of proportion to their real numbers. In any case, native influence on the folk practice of medicine was eventually eclipsed by, and mixed with, that of African practitioners.

Perhaps the worst aspect of early medicine was that many practitioners stood to gain fame, higher fees, and more patients through sheer daring. Most notorious were the numerous Spanish soldiers who, having improvised under cruel conditions of necessity, proceeded to proffer their services to the civilian population. Situated on the military crossroads of empire, some of Cuba's earliest practitioners were no doubt the rude products of such improvisation and pretention. In the absence of legitimate practitioners and unenforced professional codes, resourceful soldiers became dentists, bleeders, barbers, and surgeons, depending on the rise and fall of opportunity. A brutal anecdote will illustrate the point. In 1554, on campaign in Venezuela, soldier Diego Montes performed an "unpardonable" surgical improvisation which won him the title of El Venerable and launched him on a successful medical career. Trying to determine the nature of a serious chest wound suffered by his superior, Felipe de Utre, Montes inflicted an identical wound on an old Indian, who Montes then killed and autopsied. Armed with his new understanding of anatomy, Montes cut open and "cleaned" de Utre's chest wound, squeezing and rocking the patient in order to eject the blood that had gathered in the chest cavity. The patient miraculously survived and El Venerable began a medical career.[6]

Before 1634, but probably until much later outside of Havana, the task of licensure seems to have been flexibly interpreted by government bodies. Thus, in 1609, government officials of Santiago de Cuba, in the total absence of physicians and surgeons, named the folk healer Mariana de Nava community physician and awarded her a salary for one hundred *ducados* to maintain her residence in that city.[7] This was a considerable personal accomplishment for Mariana, first, as a woman and, second, as a *curandera*. (The next woman physician appeared — disguised as a man — in 1819.)[8] One hundred ducados was also the amount that retained the services of Licenciate Juan Tejeda de Pina when, in 1610, the Cabildo[9] found the city of Havana without the services of a physician. His obligations as the first municipal physican óf Havana were probably the same as Mariana de Nava's in Santiago: to provide medical attention to the citizens of the city and to the patients in the Hospital of Havana.[10']

Cuba's First Physician and Mutualist Plan

Before Tejeda, the few physicians who were recruited to Havana did not stay long because the prospects for making money were poor. The very first titled physician, Licenciate Gamarra, graduated from Alcalá de Henares in "all three sciences" (medicine, surgery, and pharmacy), negotiated what would seem to have been a generous contract with the Cabildo of Havana in 1559. A list of citizens, *igualados*,[11] would be provided medical care in exchange for their payment of a regular small sum, or *igula*; Gamarra would have a monopoly in Havana in the practice of medicine, surgery, and pharmacy; medicines from his pharmacy would not be covered by the *iguala*; and the remaining population, also by monopoly arrangement, would be served on a fee-for-service basis. The poor conditions of Havana are probably reflected in Gamarra's decision to abandon this arrangement in search of greater fortune elsewhere in the New World. With such difficulties, the Cabildo worked its way through the next century, at times forbidding the departure of physicians.[12]

Protophysicians and the Protomedicato

Thus, when Havana's first *protomédico* or protophysician, Francisco Muñoz de Rojas, was named in 1634, there were few legitimate practioners and scarcely any physicians to govern or defend. But the position had some value, at least for Muñoz de Rojas, for he paid the Cabildo 2,400 *reales* to occupy the office. In all probability, Muñoz de Rojas was thereby enabled to defend his own practice and also to derive income from licensure and enforcement activities aimed at other practitioners — barbers, druggists, midwives, and even improvisers and folk healers, as well as physicians and surgeons. With few wholly legitimate interests to defend, it is unlikely that complete control was ever really intended, much less achieved. The protophysician was an agent of the Royal Protomedicato, a vertically organized set of tribunals, established in the course of the sixteenth century under the Spanish crown, whose task was to carry out licensure examinations, grant practicing privileges, enforce professional codes, regulate prices of medicines and services, and defend the professions. Muñoz de Rojas served under the authority of the tribunal of the Protomedicato in Mexico City, for such a tribunal was not established in Havana until 1728, the year of the founding of the university.

After the death of Muñoz de Rojas, the post of protophysician was vacant for many years until 1709, when the Cabildo designated Francisco Teneza y Rubira to occupy the position. Like other high-ranking physicians who followed, Teneza also received a salary as administrator of the leper and municipal hospitals. Teneza, who appears to have lacked proper credentials himself, was not always successful in his more vigorous actions against deviant practitioners. Some were jailed, others fined; but at least four (the untitled and unexamined Havana physician Carlos del Rey and the druggist Vázquez, Urrutía, and Rey Bravo) were able to appeal to the Council of the Indies and gain royal concession to practice, thus circumventing the Protomedicato. When the tribunal of the Protomedicato was formed in 1728, Teneza continued to serve as its ranking member.[13]

Licensure by the Protomedicato required proof of Catholicism (purity of blood), previous study, and good character. An oral theoretical and practical examination was given, and the applicant pledged to defend the mystery of the immaculate conception, use the profession correctly, obey the laws, provide charity to the poor, give care to all possible, and to assist disciples. After the founding of the Protomedicato in Havana, all Cuban practitioners fell under its tenuous authority, and physicians who decided to practice in the interior were sometimes named protophysicians or *fiscales* (prosecutors) of the Protomedicato in their respective regions. In addition to extending the influence of the Protomedicato, the title served the physicians as an immediate legal means of professional self-defense and promised a future of influence in the distant region. Licensure frequently implied a concept of territory and enabled some practitioners to determine the conditions under which others might work — establishing fee-sharing and partnerships and yielding territory to protegés. Additionally, a physician who was also a *fiscal* of the Protomedicato could presumedly *arrest* an unauthorized competitor.[14]

Perhaps as few as six or seven legitimate practitioners were ever established in Havana before 1600, and apparently did not stay very long; perhaps fifty, mostly Spanish, arrived in the course of the seventeenth century. By the end of the eighteenth century there were some one hundred practitioners in all of Cuba.[15] These rough estimates by a Cuban medical historian include many "romance physicians," who for their deficient preparation in Latin were not, in theory, permitted to prescribe medicines without the assistance of a licensed physician.[16] By the census of 1792, such numbers would yield a ratio of one legitimate practitioner per 2,720 inhabitants, but the services of legitimate practitioners were effectively demanded by only part of the population. By another perspective, one might note that there was a ratio of one legitimate practitioner for every 1,330 whites, inasmuch as slightly more than half of the population was now black or mulatto and, of these, 60 percent were in slavery.[17] If it is true, as it is generally agreed, that the most common form of medical assistance was folk medicine or semiofficial care by phlebotomists, herbalists, and fraudulent pretenders, one may suppose that a shortage of legitimate practitioners, without great prestige anyway, was not keenly felt.

Early specialists in the pharmaceutical function, *boticarios* and *droguistas*, seem to have a largely unrecorded history. In earliest times, the physician and other practitioners performed the role of pharmacist, keeping their own storerooms of medicine and other wares. Some even advertised free consultations, charging only for medicines. In later times, the separate figure of the pharmacist often encroached upon medical practitioners. A variety of resolutions and collaboration evidently evolved from such conflict, for the partnership between relatives, physician and pharmacist, came to be formally forbidden. But pharmacy was not definitively and officially separated from medicine and the duties of the physician until the end of the eighteenth century in Spain, when under Carlos V the first *colegio*, or association, of pharmacists was formed and new regulations enacted. In Cuba, however, the old requirements of simple literacy in Latin and four years of apprenticeship with a licensed *boticario* remained in force under regulation of the Protomedicato until 1833. The popular functions of the many herbalists and charlatans of the sixteenth and seventeenth centuries were only slowly and never completely eroded from the functions of the licensed pharmacists. Of the latter, there seems to have been only three establishments in 1723 Havana, suggesting, perhaps, the preponderance of unlicensed herbalists and the role of the practitioner's storeroom.[18]

The University

The university, founded in 1734 and organized under the authority of the Franciscan order, enjoyed only marginal influence over the actual practice of medicine. With very few medical students, and a simple curriculum, most physicians were drawn from immigration. The structure of teaching, divided among three schools — theology, law and cannons, and medicine — was essentially unchanged until 1842 when the university was separated from the Franciscan monastery. The rector of the university was appointed by the bishop from the deans of the faculties, but the faculty deans were selected in an unambiguous manner. The oldest graduate was dean of the faculty, whether or not he was a member of the "cloister" of university teachers.[19] All graduates carried the title of "professor." The costume and prestige of the physician, like the lawyer, resembled that of the priest, and his degree was awarded by the highest Church official after a stately procession to the cathedral or principal church. The university was partially successful in defending Cuban medicine from new ideas and in keeping non-Spanish physicians out of Havana, where the university alone was authorized to validate foreign diplomas. The university combined secondary studies of four years for the bachelor's degree with one or two years for the degree of licenciate. After an additional year, the student could be examined for his doctorate. The licenciate was authorized to practice his profession, including teaching, while the doctorate was essentially an honorary degree.[20]

EARLY HOSPITALS

Like many early practitioners, the first hospitals were crude improvisions. Soldiers and immigrants found injury and disease. Gradually, these improvisions were institutionalized, although there was always the need to improvise against the sporadic nature of epidemic. By 1600, three cities had firmly established simple general hospitals: Santiago, Havana, and Bayamo. The following cities were not added to this list, it seems, until the eighteenth century (and then most of them late in the century): Bejucal, Guanabacoa, Jaruco, Matanzas, Puerto Príncipe, Remedios, Sancti Spíritus (today the city of Camagüey) and perhaps Trinidad. It is likely that in almost every case the general hospital was preceded by, and continued to serve as, a military hospital or infirmary. Strictly military facilities may have existed in not more than 5 or 6 other towns by 1800, but in Havana the general hospital was always supplemented by some kind of military hospital and by military infirmaries in the various fortresses and fleets.[21] In Havana and Puerto Príncipe there were small specialty hospitals for women (in Havana, beginning with four beds in 1604) and perhaps one in Trinidad before 1800. A leprosy hospital was established in Havana in 1681, and in

Puerto Príncipe in 1746. An asylum for the insane was not established until after 1800 in Havana. A few shelters near monasteries and cathedrals existed for the destitute, aged, and infirm — most of them old slaves and freedmen. In times of epidemic, emergency hospitals were set up. In Havana, there was one for sailors from 1739 to 1740, one for yellow fever from 1761 to 1762, and one for the king's slaves in 1764. Houses were rented for emergencies, as for yellow fever victims in 1763, and a Hospicio de San Isidro was also used for victims of epidemic.[22] (Although there are differences of opinion on earlier outbreaks of disease, the 1761-62 epidemic seems to have been the first occurence of yellow fever that is recognized as such by all historians. In any event, the date is significant for yellow fever did not again disappear from Havana until 1902.)[23]

The Homeless and Away-from-Home

Hospitals arose as the joint product of the etiological factors of disease and disability on the one hand and of the forces creating the homeless and away-from-home on the other: war, migration, commerce, and natural disaster. These same forces, unfortunately, greatly helped to spread, create, and expose people to disease and injury in the first place. Given the state of the healing arts, hospitals were seldom preferred, either by patient or healer, over the care of the family in the home. As in Europe, the institution of the hospital was under the auspices of the Church and served as a refuge for the homeless and away-from-home, a place, in the eyes of the Church, to seek "purification of the soul through suffering and grace through charity."[24] Just as the Roman legions had built a kind of hospital system, the armies and fleets of sixteenth century Spain organized infirmaries and gave birth to the hospital orders of friars, the brothers of San Juan de Dios, the Obregones, and the Belemitas.

Accordingly, the Hospital of Santiago de Cuba, built next to the Cathedral, was officially founded in 1522 or 1523 by Bishop Fray Juan de Úbite, following specific instructions of Emperor Charles V which were based on a 1501 Bull of Pope Alexander VI. This order institutionalized an already existing infirmary that had been improvised during Cuba's conquest by troops of Diego Velásquez from 1511 to 1520. It was here that Hernán Cortés underwent medical treatment before his departure in 1519 for Mexico. A simple thatched barracks, the infirmary-hospital was not unlike other buildings of Santiago or Havana in the first century of Spanish occupation.[25]

In early Havana, there were at least four makeshift hospitals, one known as the Rented House Hospital. The most prominent of these was built shortly before 1545 and is mentioned in the records of the Cabildo simply as "the hospital." When this building was unoccupied in 1600, it was considered the property of the Order of San Juan de Dios. As the activity of the Port of Havana increased, along with the rising numbers of forced laborers and slaves working on the city's fortifications and water supply canal, the capacity of the municipal hospital was often grossly insufficient. The governor, Juan Maldonado Barnuevo, ceded various properties to support the hospital, and at the end of the century he began the construction of a new hospital. Early hospital efforts were thus institutionalized or consolidated when the Hospital Real de San Felipe y Santiago was completed in 1599. Opened under municipal administration, it was turned over to the brothers of San Juan de Dios in 1602 and was henceforth known by the name of the religious brotherhood. With twenty initial beds, one hundred in 1664, and successive additions, particularly in 1685 and 1787, there were 400 patients, if not beds, when the hospital moved from its deteriorating location to temporary quarters above the city jail in 1861. Finally finding a new building and changing its name to Nuestra Señora de Las Mercedes in 1886, it remained Havana's only general hospital for the whole of the colonial era.[26]

The services of the friars of San Juan de Dios are indicated by the names of hospitals in Matanzas, Puerto Príncipe, Sancti Spíritus, Trinidad (?), and Villa Clara. The small women's hospital in Havana, the Hospital San Francisco de Paula, was administered by the nuns of the order of that name, as were the women's hospital in Puerto Príncipe and the later established women's hospitals in Trinidad and Villa Clara. The Belemitas founded small hospitals or convalescence homes in Havana, Bejucal, Jaruco, and two in Santiago de Cuba.[27] Other hospitals, like the Hospital de la Ermita del Cristo, suggest the influence of friars.

Hospital Finance

The money for the erection of hospitals seems to have depended greatly on the charity of the rich (which may explain why the seventeenth century, with its slow economic growth, saw little significant hospital construction) and on the treasure of the church, monasteries, and convents. The women's hospitals were such gifts of charity, the one in Havana having been founded by a rich priest and elsewhere by women of high status.[28] The first leprosy hospital (a set of native thatched houses) was financed by the wealthy don Pedro Alegre y Díaz when, in 1681, his son was ordered secluded by the authorities. Before this, there seems to have been a single large hut in an alleyway for this purpose. In 1712, a priest, Don Silvestre Alfonso, built with his own money the general hospital in Sancti Spíritus.[29]

Portions of fines and properties confiscated from law violators were sometimes designated for hospital use, but this mechanism, which dated from earliest records, hardly provided noteworthy support. More important was the similarly old and irregularly applied custom of discounting a monthly amount from each garrisoned soldier for prepayment of hospitalization and burial. In the sixteenth century, this amount was set at one *real* per month. But the separation of military from civilian hospitalization in the eighteenth century removed this source from the municipal hospital.[30]

The benefits of public or, more correctly, royal funds seem to have accrued exclusively to military hospitals and general hospitals serving both military and civilian patients. In contrast to San Juan de Dios, the well supplied military hospital of San Ambrosio was positioned within the walls of the city. But like San Juan de Dios, the late eighteenth century hospital for the king's slaves, Nuestra Señora del Pilar, was a crumbling edifice, a converted tobacco warehouse in a zone of Jesús del Monte that was periodically flooded by the stagnant waters of the water supply ditch that led to Havana from the Río Almendares.[31] Official neglect reflected the exigencies and conditions of empire, metropolis versus colony, rather than being a simple reflection of Spanish and European practice. As early as the eleventh century, peninsular hospitals attended to the mentally ill and in the early fifteenth century the first European asylum for the insane was established in Spain. But in the colony, the mentally ill were abandoned or jailed. Similarly, the colonial administration, responsible for the maintenance of the leper hospital in Havana, left it in continual disrepair.[32]

Local revenues were chronically insufficient for the support of public institutions before the nineteenth century. This fact, along with the excessive centralization in Spain of budgetary functions, greatly inhibited hospital planning. Since "public" funds were really the property of the king, the provision of such monies was indistinguishable, in principle, from the almsgiving of the rich and the Church. The viceroy, in the person of the king, was expected to be "the father of the people, the patron of monasteries and hospitals, the protector of the poor, and particularly of the widows and orphans of the conquerors, and the old servants of the king, all of whom would suffer were it not for the relief afforded them by the viceroy."[33] But the viceroy was distant, in Mexico City, and his closest representative was the Audiencia of Santo Domingo. Thus it was the cabildo, greatly dependent on local revenue, that shouldered the immediate responsibility for hospitals and public sanitation, while a bishop and cathedral was not established in Havana until late in the eighteenth century. A marked change occurred when Cuba became a captaincy-general in 1777, for the role of the captain-general was essentially the same as that of a viceroy. At the same time, economic expansion gave the Cuban colony its first financial self-sufficiency.

Division of Labor

Occupational categories in the hospital were simple: a barber-surgeon, steward, chaplain, servants, and perhaps a visiting physician. As in

Table 2.1
Positions and Monthly Salaries Before and
After Reorganization of San Ambrosio Hospital, 1793*

Before		After	
Positions	Pesos	Positions	Pesos
Inspector	—	Inspector	—
Controller	35	Controller	35
Head Chaplain	30	Chaplain	30
2nd Chaplain	30	Scribe	18
3rd Chaplain and Translator		Majordomo	30
(*Ideomas*)	22½	Head Intern in Medicine	30
Commissary of Entrance	18	Head Surgeon	40
Scribe	18	2nd Surgeon	40
Majordomo	22	Head Intern in Surgery	25
Head Physician	50	Head Nurse	20
2nd Physician	25	4 Interns @ 10 ea.	40
3rd Physician	40	4 Ward Attendants @ 10 ea.	40
Head Intern (*Practicante*)		Launderer	20
in Medicine	30	Dispensor	18
Head Surgeon	40	Porter	18
2nd Surgeon	40	Cook	12
3rd Surgeon	40	23 Forced Servants	—
Head Intern in Surgery	30		
Head Nurse	20	Total: 45 personnel	
7 Interns (*Practicantes*)			
@ 12 ea.	84	Pesos: 416	
7 Ward Attendants (*Cavos de*			
Sala) @ 12 ea.	84		
Medical Inspector or			
Inspector of Medicines			
(*Insp. de Med.*)	12		
Launderer	12		
Dispensor	12		
Bleeder	12		
Porter	12		
Head Cook	16		
2nd Cook	4		
40 Forced Servants (slaves)	—		

Total: 78 personnel

Pesos: 728½

*Data are derived from Luis A. de Arce, "El Real Hospital Nuestra Señora del Pilar en el siglo XVIII (un hospital para los esclavos del Rey), 1764-1793," *Cuadernos de Historia de Salud Pública*, no. 41, Havana: Ministerio de Salud Pública, 1969, pp. 64-66.

Europe, the pragmatic consequence of the homely role of the woman and of the hospital was that wherever civilian workers were available, many services were provided by older women, called *madres*, with authority and duties that went with their suggestive title. In a few hospitals, late in the period, these women were irregularly joined by their wealthy counterparts seeking grace through acts and gifts of charity. Sometimes these functions were performed by nuns, and the priest must have been a not uncommon figure. Friars and other men served as male attendants. Though often disobedient, friars and nuns were forbidden to act as medical practitioners;[34] medical intervention was ostensibly performed by barbers, surgeons, and physicians, depending on their availability, which, as we have seen, was not great. Prescription of drugs was theoretically the exclusive province of the latter. Teaching was an insignificant and informal activity in the hospital until after 1800. Teachers at the university, however, sometimes held hospital posts and were likely accompanied by a student who may have also gained a hospital position. Similarly, a student was required to practice one year under a licensed physician before being examined for licensing by the Protomedicato or its subdelegates.

In sharp contrast to the improverished municipal hospital and the hospital for the king's slaves was the San Ambrosio military hospital. Replacing or expanding from its original site, a mansion next to the Hospicio de San Isidro donated for the purpose by the bishop in 1744, San Ambrosio was the first hospital construction which reflected the beginnings of great sugar wealth in Cuba and also the age of endemic yellow fever, the scourge of new soldiers and immigrants. With such attention at the end of the long prelude to the first medical revolution, the salaried offices of San Ambrosio soon became Cuba's first medical bureaucracy, its positions being held by Havana's most influential physicians. When the patients and staff of the woeful Nuestra Señora del Pilar were transferred to San Ambrosio in 1793, the bureaucracy was reviewed and severely reduced, as the Table 2.1 suggests.

San Ambrosio's expansion to 400 beds meant a mixed group of patients. Near the new, but "provisional," quarters for sick slaves and convicts from Nuestra Señora del Pilar were wards which served military officers, and civilians and clergy of high rank. Another ward was special for victims of the white plague or tuberculosis. The reorganization of San Ambrosio suggests a decline in the position of physicians compared to surgeons and tended to improve the meager salaries of such essential low-ranking personnel as launderers, dispensors, porters, and cooks. The physicians who disappeared from the payroll (some transferred to other posts in Havana) included the most prestigious: Don Nicolás del Valle, who became the protophysician of Havana, and Don Lorenzo Hernández, who held a professorship at the university. (His student, Thomás Romay, began a hospital appointment at this time and later served for many years as head physician.) The steward, Don Antonio Bretos, not only survived the reorganization, but his wife continued to receive 128 pesos per month as rent on five houses owned by her in the vicinity of the hospital, a practice that was continued for at least sixty years. Located near the early university, San Ambrosio and the Hospicio de San Isidro would soon be the logical sites for hospital courses in medical education.[36]

Specialization of hospitals or within hospitals followed a small number of social and medical categories. Hospitalization was, first of all, almost exclusively directed to the homeless and the away-from-home because the home was clearly preferred as the location for the sick bed. A consequence of this preference was that there was little significant hospital specialization for wealthy patients, simply because they did not present themselves for hospitalization. Even when away from home, the rich found a sick bed in homes or hospices which could be privately hired. Only slowly did this practice come to be regarded as hospitalization, while the provision of such shelter by medical and lay entrepreneurs grew to significant dimensions, particularly in Havana and its nearby towns.

The social and demographic categories which did influence hospital specialization were the following (listed in order of their appearance in Cuban hospital history): officer and common soldier, military and civilian, white and black, slave (or convict) and free, male and female, and adult and child. Medical characteristics which figured in hospital specialization may be summarized in the following dichotomies: (1) conditions requiring clinical treatment versus those requiring simple asylum, (2) contagious or dangerous versus noncontagious or innocuous conditions, and (3) somatic versus psychological conditions.

Soldiers were the first to stimulate hospital services; hence the first social category of specialization was the division between officers and conscripts. The arrival of poor immigrants and forced laborers (slaves and convicts) next required separate wards or hospitals. Somewhat later the needs of women, particularly those who were homeless in late pregnancy, excited public and charitable beneficence. On the heels of women came the children; foundling homes and orphanages appeared in the eighteenth century.

The first military hospitals separated, after the fashion of the existing Spanish model, the functions of asylum and clinical treatment. These elementary divisions later appeared in other social categories. Separate wards for contagious disease appeared first in military hospitals. Cholera victims came to be isolated in separate, often makeshift buildings. And lepers, always outcast (at least the poor), were forced into "hospitals" when their numbers grew sufficient to cause alarm. Here there were sometimes separate quarters for blacks, but there was sexual comingling. (When provisions were insufficient, the lepers only weapon was to threaten to invade the town.) Hospitalization for the dangerous "insane" only occurred when jails proved insufficient. If there were facilities for blacks and convicts, the insane were introduced as well. But it is unlikely that black women found their way to women's hospitals, while aged, incapacitated, and destitute blacks found only one or two institutional shelters.

These tendencies of early hospital specialization hold not only for Havana, but also for Santiago and Camagüey, towns which developed similar ranges of services by 1800, although not at the same pace or under the same pressures as Havana.[37]

The provisional nature of many services and the shortage in Cuba of religious personnel probably explain the tendency of Cuban hospitals to be somewhat more medical and less like hostels or hospices than their European counterparts. Strong military association, less substantial internal migration and commercial travel, and few parish churches and cathedrals would support such a difference. A shortage of beds would also limit the "hotel" function. If the one hundred beds of Havana's San Juan de Dios had the thoroughly unlikely turnover of seven hundred patients per month in 1668 and an average length of stay of 4.3 days,[38] calculated at maximum efficiency, there was abundant patient demand in relation to the services available.

However, aside from psychological and physical comfort, early hospitals and practitioners made insignificant overall contribution to the general level of health and well-being. Given the state of medical technology, one may find at least as many instances where early services were detrimental as instances where they were beneficial to the well-being of the patient and society. Blood letting, often in great excess, was the preferred treatment for fevers. Surgery bred infection and hospitals were correctly avoided as sources of disease.[39] This is not to say, of course, that early services did not serve important, indeed indispensable, social functions or that there were not significant numbers of practitioners who helped more than they harmed. But on the whole, the development of various medical practitioners and hospitals is less a history of intervention against disease than a testament to the great need and the resourcefulness of those who developed approximations of health care for different population strata of Cuba. With little knowledge or effective implementation of public hygiene, the early state of health in Cuba is best seen as an unhindered product of the economy and of the ecology of disease.

ECONOMY AND LIVING CONDITIONS

To make a point that will not be belabored elsewhere, the worst conditions of the early period, indeed throughout the whole of pre-republican history, are associated with assaults on human dignity and freedom: the conquest and forced labor of the native population and the forced immigration and enslavement of Africans. The conditions of the latter varied by type of industry and technology, and these factors changed greatly in the course of Cuban history. Health conditions also varied between city and country, with the former subject to epidemics that accompanied sea trade and commerce. Conditions also varied considerably by social class. The wealthy were better housed, better fed, and enjoyed better water supplies.[40] Often the rich would flee the cities in time of epidemic and take up lodging in a country estate, a privileged complement to the irregular effectiveness of quarantine, which was employed as early as 1711 in Havana.[41] The colonial era ended in an orgy of disease, starvation, and disability that was the last great cost of empire to the Spanish and the tragic price of liberty for Cuba.

Slow Early Development

The exclusive existence of hospitals in three cities of Cuba during the first two centuries of Spanish occupation reflects the slow development of the island. After initial mining and agricultural experiments failed (wheat, grapes, and olives did poorly), little official attention was given to the goals of developing the interior. Instead, as Spain passed over Cuba, the structure of the island's society grew upon the role of large and secure harbors in the gold-laden empire. The provisioning of merchant fleets, which often waited long periods before the protected voyage to Spain, and their military defenders, created versatile traders and small repair, shipbuilding, and food processing industries. The interior responded with cattle for jerked beef, the staple of the seaman's (and slave's) diet, as well as hides, for a long time the chief Cuban export. Salted vegetables and dried fruit were provided, along with secondary exports: tobacco, sugar, and fine woods.

Population growth was slow, increasing towards the end of the period. The sixteenth century average was not more than 1,500 Spanish immigrants per year to all parts of the empire. By 1775 the population had finally reached 170,000, but this was helped by the forced immigration of more than 60,000 African slaves before 1760 and at least 90,000 by 1798.[42] In 1775 roughly 40 percent of the population were black or mulatto, of whom two-thirds were slaves. Of the slaves, about one-third were women, indicating their recent African origin. The census of 1775 found 44 percent of the population concentrated in Havana province, and in 1760 Havana itself was the third largest city of the hemisphere after Lima and Mexico. On the whole, the slowly growing economy enjoyed a stability which, thanks to a variety of native foods, provided a substantial, if often contaminated, diet.

The early contrast, a small population with two cosmopolitan cities, led to the rise of a kind of urbanized landed gentry who, living off the land, resided in the walled cities. Since the offices of the Cabildo of Havana were sold to the highest bidder after the sixteenth century, they became the almost hereditary property of this class of landowners.

Land was available for the asking until the 1730s and cheap until the end of the century. A few peasant farmers, some escaped slaves and Indians, produced native products: yucca, maize, avocado, sweet potatoes, beans, pumpkins, medicinal plants, and a little tobacco. These products were also grown for consumption and urban sale on the more or less self-sufficient ranches, sugar plantations, and tobacco farms. In the early eighteenth century, the partial ascendency of tobacco stimulated new settlement near the ports of Trinadad, Bayamo, Manzanillo, and the areas of Vuelta Abajo, Holguín, Yara, and Güines. These developments, the effort at monopoly by the King's Tobacco Company, conflict between tobacco farmers and cattlemen, and the garrisoning of tobacco areas against contraband and rebellion led to the establishment of the few small eighteenth century hospitals in the interior. Sugar, produced in Cuba since 1520, numbered in the mid-eighteenth century perhaps one hundred small mills covering 10,000 acres, with a yearly export of some five hundred tons.[43]

Ranches and tobacco farms offered the most favorable work conditions for slaves; the former demanded long periods of unsupervised work, and the labor demanded by the latter was constant, intensive, and tedious but not back-breaking. By contrast, sugar mills and plantations provided the greatest hardship, but here, as in ranches and *tabacales*, slaves lived in village-like clusters of huts and were allowed to keep gardens and even sell their produce. The self-sufficiency in food of early agricultural units was an extremely important health-related factor, helping to secure a fresh and balanced supply of food and to protect laborers from prevailing market and credit instabilities.[44]

Slavery

Depending on the distance to respectable authorities, Spanish and Roman law regulating slavery had some effect on property rights, legal personalities, birth, marriage, and burial rights, and the right of *coartación*. A slave could live under conditions of virtual freedom after paying a specified installment or *coartación* on his total value. Slaves could also be given their freedom. The large numbers of freedmen who established themselves in the urban trades suggest that these processes worked to some degree. But suicide was common throughout the whole of the slavery era, inspired by the severity of conditions and by the belief that after death one would return to Africa. To protect the health of his slaves, the plantation owner in this early era was unlikely to employ a Spanish surgeon or barber, but gave African folk healers freedom and encouragement to practice their arts. To aid morale, if not health, a sugar mill would include a distillery to manufacture *aguardiente*. The Church tended to support, though without great vigor, the enforcement of slavery codes and determined that the slaves should receive elementary religious instruction and sacraments. Meat on Fridays, work on Sundays, and burial in unconsecrated cemeteries were banned. One important Church policy, with origins in the sixteenth century occupation of Peru, was the encouragement of African religious organizations and a blend of Christianity. Vigorously promoted in mid-eighteenth century Cuba by bishop Monsignor Morell de Santa Cruz, this policy probably lessened the psychological and cultural disruption under slavery.[45]

Slaves who lived in the cities were considered to have better working conditions than those in agriculture. Here the compliance with slavery codes was thought to be greater and the style of life more relaxed. But urban slaves faced greater exposure to epidemic diseases of the city. In contrast to the lofty position of household slaves, the most unhealthy conditions may have been experienced by the king's slaves. Since they were builders and maintainers of public works and fortifications of the city, or workers in the king's tobacco factory, they lived regimented in barracks, afflicted by every contagious disease. So grievous were their conditions that special arrangements were always made for sick slaves, as in 1761 when a special hospital for victims of yellow fever was improvised *adjoining* the Royal Tobacco Factory.[46]

The real test of the moral order of slavery was the treatment of old slaves and others incapacitated for work, while between eight and ten percent of the working slave population had to be replaced each year.[47] Writing at the end of the eighteenth century, Licenciate Francisco Barrera y Domingo describes one fate of aged slaves and *emancipados* in Havana:

> Besides keeping their children as slaves they [the masters] abandon the father and mother, even throwing them out of the house, so that they die, as they do every day, full of misery, naked, made into skeletons, underneath the *Arco de Belén*, which is the resting place for these unfortunates, in payment for having been slaves for twenty-five or thirty years. Note: *Belén* is a convent for the *padres Belemitas*, where every day they give two good meals to the poor; here is where the archways are, full of *miserables*, who, being slaves, do not go to the Hospital, because they don't want to take them and here is where almost every day they die.[48]

Life and death in Cuba was but the last step in a complicated dehumanizing chain of events. Passage from Africa was infamous for its high mortality, and the mortality rate in African capture, concentration, and preparation for sale may have been even greater. Upon arrival in Cuba, the slaves, weakened by the preceeding experience and kept in barracks near the waterfront, were set upon by whatever plague happened to be attacking the population in Havana. And, as if in fair exchange, the slaves communicated new exotic diseases to the Havana residents.

Fearing the political consequences of a large slave population, the Spanish never permitted Cuba to become a garrison state of masters and slaves, at least not as early or to the same degree as in the nearby French, English, and Dutch islands. At the same time, reflecting this Spanish policy, the small scale of early plantations, average a mere thirty eight acres in the early seventeenth century, prevented extreme regimentation on the plantation level. The long period of relatively unthreatened and mildly enlightened paternalism created conditions that prevailed until the last half of the eighteenth century for the development of an Afro-Cuban culture and the movement of mulattoes and blacks into the free labor force, into some of the professions, and even into positions of modest wealth. The early period set a foundation, then, for an Afro-Cuban society.[49]

The long early period must also be regarded as the real base of the health system that emerged in future years. The eighteenth and nineteenth century universities were more alike than different. Indeed some of the earliest patterns are still predominant in the presocialist university of 1958. A similar comment would apply to the profession itself — which has never completely given up its severe clinical eye and mysterious aloofness — and also to certain patterns of hospital development. The early rented houses are precursory to the *quintas* and *casas de salud* and the earliest *iguala* anticipates mutualism. Finally, the medicine of early Cuba long survived in the folk medicine practiced among the rural and less privileged sectors (though not limited to them) of Cuba.[50]

NOTES

1. Postmortem caesarian section was infrequently performed until the eighteenth century when it was urged by the Church and instructed by the king; see Aristides A. Moll, *Aesculapius in Latin America* (Philadelphia: W.B. Saunders, 1944), pp. 163-64. The native Siboneys were known to practice the operation; see José A. Martínez-Fortún y Foyo, "Apuntes para la historia de la odontología en Cuba," *Cuadernos de Historia de Salud Pública, no. 23*, (Havana: Ministerio de Salud Pública, 1963), p. 11.

2. Martíñez-Fortún y Foyo, pp. 11-13.

3. Mario del Pino y de la Vega, "Apuntes para la historia de los hospitales de Cuba (1523 a 1899)," *Cuadernos de historia de Salud Pública, no. 24*, (Havana: Ministerio de Salud Pública, 1963), p. 22.

4. Ibid.

5. Ibid., p. 24.

6. Ibid., p. 21. See also Ambrosio Perera, *Historia de la medicina en Venezuela* (Caracas: Ministerio de Sanidad y Asistencia Social, Imprenta Nacional, 1951), pp. 17-20.

7. del Pino y de la Vega, p. 21. See also María Julia de Laura, "Laura Martínez de Carvajal y del Camino (primera graduada de medicina en Cuba) en el septuagésimo quinto aniversario de su graduación (15 de julio de 1889)," *Cuadernos de Historia de la Salud Pública, no. 28*, (Havana: Ministerio de Salud Pública, 1964), pp. 94-97. Taking mild exception to the view of this author, it may be argued that Mariana de Nava should be remembered as the first officially recognized woman physician in Cuba. Her actual lack of university credentials or proper examination is indistinguishable, in principle, from the same lack of credentials of male practitioners who, from time to time, enjoyed official and even high medical status.

8. For an account of Cuba's first university trained and officially licensed woman physician, Enriqueta Faber, see Emilio Roig de Leuchsenring, *Médicos y medicina en Cuba: Historia, Biografía, Costumbrismo* (Havana: Museo Historico de las Ciencias Médicas "Carlos J. Finlay," 1965), pp. 31-49.

9. The term *cabildo* has referred to a variety of councils, meetings, clubs, associations, or chapters. The cabildo or *gobierno* of an average town might have included "six *regidores*, or aldermen, and two *alcaldes*, or justices, elected by regidores each year." In early settlements, the council sometimes was formed spontaneously by elections and other means, but offices were soon inherited or purchased as in Spain. See Edward Gaylord Bourne, *Spain in America, 1450-1580*, first published in 1904 (New York: Barnes and Noble, 1962), p. 236.

10. Roig de Leuchsenring, pp. 23-24.

11. The word *igualado* is a participial noun derived from the verb *igualar* or *igualarse*, which may mean to make equal, one with another, or to reach an accord or agreement. This term, along with the related noun *iguala* (which seems to be specific to medical contracts) also found use in the language of mutualist medical plans of the nineteenth and twentieth centuries in Spain and America.

12. del Pino y de la Vega, p. 19, and Roig de Leuchsenring, pp. 21-22.

13. Emeterio S. Santovenia, "El protomédico de la Habana," *Cuadernos de Historia Sanitaria, no. 1*, (Havana: Ministerio de Salubridad y Asistencia Social, 1952), pp. 18-61. Also see Manuel García Hernández and Susan Martínez-Fortún y Foyo, "Apuntes históricos relativos a la farmacia en Cuba," *Cuadernos de Salud Pública, no. 33*, (Havana: Ministerio de Salud Pública, 1967), p. 14.

14. Roig de Leuchsenring, p. 36.

15. Martínez-Fortún y Foyo, pp. 11-12.

16. Moll, pp. 115-18.

17. See discussion of the census of 1791 and 1792 in Hugh Thomas, *Cuba: The Pursuit of Freedom* (New York: Harper and Row, 1971), pp. 91-92. The numbers were:

Total population	272,301
Whites	133,559
Mulatto or Negro	138,742
Free	54,142
Slave	84,590

18. García Hernández and Martínez-Fortún y Foyo, p. 15.

19. Luis Felipe LeRoy y Gálvez, "Dr. Juan M. Sánchez de Bustamente y García del Barrio," *Cuadernos de Historia de Salud Pública, no. 42*, (Havana: Ministerio de Salud Pública, 1969), p. 103.

20. Yet a student who earned his *bachillerato* could be licensed by the Protomedicato after two years of practice with a physician. In the 114 years under Franciscan direction (1728-1824) only ninety-one physicians graduated with advanced titles of licenciate or doctor. The distinguishing feature of the doctorate was the writing of a thesis, usually a short monograph. See Luis F. LeRoy, "Los origenes de los estudios universitarios de las ciencias médicas en Cuba," *Revista "Finlay" de Historia Sanitaria* 7 (July-December 1966): 46.

21. These data are adopted from del Pino y de la Vega, pp. 43-46.

22. Ibid., pp. 38-39.

23. Foreshadowing the cruel end of the nineteenth century, the English troops that captured Havana in 1762 lost more than one-third of their number to disease or 4,708, along with 1,300 seamen and marines, not including figures for slave losses. See Thomas, p. 48.

24. Ray H. Elling, "The Hospital's Changing Position in the Community," manuscript, p. 4.

25. del Pino y de la Vega, pp. 26-28.

26. Ibid., pp. 28-34; and Guillermo Lage, "El primer hospital de la Habana," *Cuadernos de Historia Sanitaria, no. 3,* (Havana: Ministerio de Salubridad y Asistencia Social, 1952), pp. 40-41.

27. Ibid., p. 44.

28. Ibid.

29. Ibid.

30. Guillermo Lage, pp. 36-40.

31. See Luis A. de Arce, "El Real Hospital Nuestra Señora del Pilar en el siglo XVIII (un hospital para los esclavos del Rey), 1764-1793," *Cuadernos de Historia de Salud Pública, no. 41* (Havana: Ministerio de Salud Pública, 1969), p. 93.

32. For a discussion of the early care of leprosy victims and the "insane," see del Pino y de la Vega, pp. 35-37 and pp. 39-41, respectively.

33. Advice of the departing (fourth) Viceroy of New Spain, Martín de Enríquez, cited in Bourne, pp. 229-30.

34. del Pino y de la Vega, pp. 20-21. This practice dated far into the Middle Ages, as convents and monasteries served as places of learning and succor. Controversy emerged over the charging of fees.

35. de Arce, pp. 64-66.

36. These courses were formally begun under the leadership of Tomás Romay after 1800.

37. René Ibañez Varona, "Historia de los hospitales y asilos de Puerto Príncipe de Camagüey (período colonial)," *Cuadernos de Historia Sanitaria, no. 6,* (Havana: Ministerio de Salubridad y Asistencia Social, 1954). The Camagüey experience is worth noting for comparison. Although its civilian population was substantial, it developed no hospital until around 1725, for the city lacked military and commercial travelers. After attacks by pirates and escaped slaves, the military garrison was increased. This stimulated the construction of a general hospital with separate services for soldiers, white civilians, and blacks; each of these services was divided into acute and chronic *(asilo)* wards. A woman's hospital was begun but never used until the nineteenth century, when a separate military hospital was built and a foundling home established. Lepers enjoyed a small refuge on a remote ranch until 1731 when a new refuge was built, designating the old one for use by blacks and slaves. Before

this move, the lepers threatened to invade the town if they did not receive improved food and facilities.

38. del Pino y de la Vega, p. 34, citing José A. Martínez-Fortún y Foyo, *Cronología de la medicina cubana, 1492-1800* (Havana: 1947), p. 20. My calculation of 4.3 days per patient assumes full occupancy and hence the real average stay, if the data are correct, would be smaller. The occupancy, however, for the month indicated could have been greater, however, than 100 percent. While this would mean a longer average stay, it would similarly indicate a high demand for hospitalization.

39. Thus the services rendered in a hospital were intrinsically charitable, for those who served risked contagion; sometimes admired, they were also held at a distance by the general population.

40. For a discussion of these conditions, see "Finlay's Early Work," in chapter 4. The rich were supplied by cisterns and wells; the poor often took their water from open canals. Until the mid-nineteenth century, Havana's water was largely supplied by the Zanja Real, an open canal (with many outlet branches) from the Almendares River at a point eight kilometers distant from the city. See Elena López Serrano, "Apuntes para la historia: ingeniería sanitaria," *Revista Cubana de Administración de Salud* 2 (July-September 1976) 3: 307-19.

41. Moll, p. 76.

42. Apparently a modest estimate offered by Hubert H. S. Aimes, *A History of Slavery in Cuba, 1511-1868* (New York, 1907), p. 269, cited by Thomas, p. 95.

43. Thomas, p. 61.

44. For a description of early enterprises, see Thomas, p. 29 and p. 35.

45. Ibid., pp. 39-40. However, the role of the Church, says Thomas, was not on the whole progressive. A good review of literature on this subject (cultural and religious influences on the institution of slavery), along with a similar dim view, is found in Franklin W. Knight, *Slave Society in Cuba During the Nineteenth Century* (Madison, Wisconsin: University of Wisconsin Press, 1970), pp. xv-xix.

46. Evidently, improvised quarters for soldiers and slaves were established in buildings (probably warehouses) adjoining the Royal Tobacco Factory in 1761 and 1764. Institutionalized as Nuestra Señora del Pilar, the environs of the factory (and after 1827, the factory itself) served as an "overflow" facility for the nearby San Ambrosio Military Hospital and the Hospicio de San Isidro. See del Pino y de la Vega, pp. 38-39 and de Arce, pp. 10-13.

47. These estimates have varied greatly, but the rate seems to have been lower in earlier times. Julio Le Riverend suggests as few as 3% in near 1750 and 5%-8% in the mid 1800s. See his *Economic History of Cuba*, translated by M. J. Cazabón and Homero León (Havana: Book Institute, 1967), p. 158. Estimates by Knight seem to be lower; those of Thomas, for the first half of the 19th century, higher, at the figures given here. See: Knight, p. 82 and Thomas, p. 170.

48. Francisco Barrera Domingo, *Reflexiones Históricas Físico Naturales Médico Quirúrgicas* (Havana: Ediciones C.R., 1953), p. 156, cited by del Pino y de la Vega, p. 37.

49. See Thomas, who elaborates this point, pp. 159-167.

50. In presocialist Cuba, as elsewhere in Latin America, the medical journey from the cosmopolitan services of urban elites to the folk services of the hinterland was a journey also in time. See Roemer, "Medical Care and Social Class in Latin America."

3
The First
Medical Revolution,
1790-1830

TOMAS ROMAY Y CHACON

The substance of the first medical revolution in Cuba is reflected in the life of one of its prominent agents, the physician and encyclopedist, Tomás Romay y Chacón. An examination of Romay's life unearths at once the changes in the health system and the closely related socioeconomic dynamics of the period. A leader in public health and medical education, Romay found support in the exclusive Sociedad Económica de Amigos del País, a group whose great influence derived in turn from the spiral of agricultural wealth that was the constant object of the society's labors. The economic developments of this period from 1790 to 1830 (and extending on either side) transformed the rather placid paternalism of early urban and agricultural Cuba into a brutal and cosmopolitan slavocracy of huge proportions. Like the economy, which jumped forward after being loosened from a long period of colonial constraints, the health system responded to new domestic conditions and to forces that had been accumulating in Europe during the past century. While the ensuing changes were not earthshaking, they were highly significant precursory events to the really earthshaking changes in the health system that occur at the end of the nineteenth century.

Romay's work included teaching reform, introduction and propagation of smallpox vaccination, public sanitation, the protection of slaves, regulation of pharmacies, encouragement of European immigration, land reform, and town development. While his role was decidedly modern for its eclectic view of medical science and broad concern for living conditions as relevant to health, Romay's ideas and work were constrained by the om-

41

nipresent institution of plantation slavery that came to dominate Cuban society in his lifetime. The growth of plantation economy propelled the significant changes in living conditions that shaped the health status of the island and, at the same time, financed the elementary public health inadequately, in preventive medicine, the effectiveness of curative dimensions of medicine remained rather unchanged. The economic context, it bears repeating, was indeed revolutionary, generating new demands and problems, new resources, new orientations, and also new constraints for the Cuban health endeavor.

Here I have chosen to first discuss Romay's family, class, and economic roots, his public role and attitude toward slavery, and his work in support of white population development. Having thus set the larger socioeconomic context, I will then treat the work that was Romay's central contribution to health promotion: the organization of smallpox vaccination, the reorganization of medical education, hospital administration, and the control of fraudulent medicines.

FAMILY, CLASS, AND ECONOMIC ROOTS

Tomás Romay y Chacón (1764-1849) was born not far from the hospital San Juan de Dios in a wealthy suburban expansion of the old city of Havana.[1] His parents were representative of rising social classes. Tomás's father, Don Lorenzo Romay, was a man of the "better" class in Havana, an entrepreneur of sorts, son of an infantry lieutenant but certainly not a member of the central oligarchy. Don Lorenzo was the owner of several houses in Havana inherited by his mother. The fact that Lorenzo's brother, Fray Pedro, was a teacher in the Convento de Predicadores (where Tomás was tutored), probably indicates the purity of the elder Romay's Catholic background back to at least four generations.[2] Lorenzo, in any case, managed with María de los Angeles Valdés Chacón to marry into the heart of the landed Cuban aristocracy. The Chacón family, holders of original royal land grants of the early seventeenth century, had at least one immediate family member, Laureano Chacón, in the Cabildo of Havana in the 1760s. He was elected, in fact, to be one of the two mayors of Havana in 1762. In keeping with tightly intermarried creole aristocracy, Laureano Chacón's brother-in-law, the Marqués de Villalta, happened also to be a member of the Cabildo.[3]

Recently, the landed aristocracy from which Romay's mother was born had begun to turn part of their cattle estates to sugar production. Owing to high interest rates of 20 to 30 percent on money and credit extended by merchants (for there were no general banks in Cuba until late in the nineteenth century), the Cubans who were best able to profit from the rising sugar market were the already wealthy landowners. Only they could begin with the necessary ingredients: vast areas of virgin land to plant as old land wore out, forests to cut for buildings and as fuel for the boiling cauldrons, cattle and oxen to run machinery and feed slaves, and sometimes the cash to buy slaves — the most costly and restrictive factor of sugar production. Everyone except the very richest landowners, or those who were also merchants, had to rely on credit and thus only the largest could ever hope to be free from debt. One of the richest mill owners was Romay's grandmother and godmother, María Teresa Chacón, the Marquesa de Casa Bayona, who was one of the eight planters who owned a sugar mill producing more than one hundred tons in 1761, on the eve of a great upsurge in Cuban sugar.[4] In that year, the English capture of Havana gave new freedoms, ideas, and credits to the elements of the Cuban oligarchy and merchant class who determined to enrich themselves on the explosive potential of Cuban sugar in an expansive international market. For old Cuba, the great reserves of virgin land contrasted ominously with the already maximized and soon declining planting in the small English, French, and Dutch island colonies.

The future director of the medical revolution was therefore nourished from the most opportune union of the time-aspiring merchant entrepreneur and established but expansionist aristocracy. While some portions of the old landed aristocracy declined, usually by indebtedness, successful new families bought titles of nobility and often married into families of the central oligarchy. One such family was the González-Alvarez Guillén family, into which Tomás Romay married in 1796, gaining a wife and two very influential brothers-in-law.[5] Romay himself came to possess sugar lands and slaves and gained the title of "physician to the royal family."

From a family of slave owners, the institution of slavery was never an abstract or remote concept in Romay's early years. Considering that there had been no fundamental technological improvements since the roller mill was devised in fifteenth century Sicily, the increase from an average of thirty or so tons of sugar to over one hundred tons in the Chacón mill was purely the product of a painful increase in scale and the employment of some one hundred slaves. (The relationship was constant over many years: one slave produced one ton of sugar.)[6] Romay's mother was probably assisted by household slaves, and when Romay passed for secondary studies to the somber halls of the Real Seminario de San Carlos y San Ambrosio, that devout institution owned two large sugar mills and many slaves.[7] In these formative years, the slave trade became highly visible in Havana, and by the time Romay finished his studies at the Real y Pontífica Universidad de San Ambrosio y de La Habana, some fifty thousand new slaves were sold in Cuba (1763-1793), almost all of them at the port of Havana and almost as many as in the two preceding centuries.[8] The king imported slaves to improve the fortifications of the city, sugar mills multiplied, and the United States, a rising new nation of slave traders and consumers of sugar, rum, and molasses, gained its independence.

The Papel Periódico and the Sociedad Económica

After two years of private practice under the physician Dr. Manuel Sacramento, Romay, in 1791, gained his medical license by *oposición* (a public oral examination before a tribunal) from the Royal Protomedicato and, also by *oposición*, in the area of pathology, he obtained the title of doctor from the University in 1793. In the same year Romay emerged in public life as a founder of the *Papel Periódico*, Cuba's first newspaper.[9] His collaboration on the *Papel* indicates an early association with two of his most famous contemporaries: the enterprising economist-businessman-planter married into the O'Farrill family, Francisco de Arango (1765-1839) and the liberal captain-general-mill owner and brother-in-law of the Conde de O'Reilly, Luis de Las Casas y Aragorri (1745-1807). It is in the pages of the *Papel Periódico* that Romay began the open polemic against narrow scholasticism in the medical school. His writings on matters relating to health, especially the promotion of smallpox vaccination after 1804, helped to make the *Papel* the first organ of public health propaganda in Cuba.

Also in 1793, Romay joined the same group of luminaries in the foundation of the Sociedad Económica de Amigos del País, an ingenious mix of college, board of inquiry, and social club. The society developed intellectual resources, participated in government, and expressed the central interests of the entrepreneurial classes at home and in the halls of Spanish and foreign governments. Prominent among the projects of the society were public schools, hospitals, asylums, a poorhouse, roads, bridges, a public library and an aqueduct for Havana. Here Romay served as president of the sections on education and medical sciences, as a member of the Inspección General de Estudios and of the Junta Superior de Sanidad. Romay's name also appears as secretary for various activities of the Junta de Fomento (Arango's development board), the Real Consulado (a kind of informational and investigative body) and the society itself. Finally in 1842, four years before his death, Romay gained the highest position of the society, director, succeeding his eminent son-in-law, José de la Luz y Caballero.[10]

The public works, and the first financial self-sufficiency of the colonial government, were made possible by a phenomenal stage of economic growth that was the real objective of the society. Here the resourceful members of the society were aided, if not entirely propelled, by powerful new forces: the collapse of Haitian (St. Domingue) sugar after the successful slave rebellion of 1791, the decline of Jamaica, the expansion of the North American market, and the doubling of European sugar prices hastened by the European wars of the French Revolutionary and Napoleonic periods. To such events were soon added the destruction of the Spanish fleet at Trafalgar, the abdication of a king to Napoleon, intermittent civil war, the imposition of a liberal Spanish constitution in 1812, and rebellion throughout the far-flung empire. Under liberal captain-generals, Cuba lived in a state of near independence which was exploited by the Cuban upper classes, not for political independence, but for self-enrichment.

The result for Cuba was a barrage of economc activity that had profound social and human dimensions. In the Havana area alone, 179 new mills were built between 1792 and 1806.[11] Matanzas, the first province and port city east of Havana, was developed. Great reserves of the king's hardwood forests and the marginally less profitable tobacco farms of Havana province were burned to make way for sugar, and ship building tradesmen turned to sugar-related work. However, in the midst of overall growth, interest rates remained high while the chronic instabilities of market and production frequently caused ruin for small planters and even for large planters who became overextended. As Hugh Thomas has observed, a process emerged which at once enriched and destroyed much of the old aristrocracy, while new families, many of whom had gained their new cash reserves by direct participation in the slave trade, emerged as respectable and prominent members of the sugar-slavery oligarchy.[12]

ROMAY AND SLAVERY

Both the human physical dimension of economic expansion are suggested in the statistics of slave imports (see Table 3.1).

The economic tendencies which appeared in the 1760s escalated in the 1790s and skyrocketed after the turn of the century. The experiment of 1789 in free trade in slaves was made general in 1804 and slaves became available in numbers which, for the first sustained period, approached the demands of planters. Ironically, the 1807 abolition of direct English participation in the slave trade probably increased the sale of slaves. A similar effect followed the English-influenced Spanish announcement in 1817 that all traffic in slaves would be abolished in 1821. An aggressive expansion of British industry and commerce augered weakly for enforcement but strongly for the nonenforcement of anti-slavery agreements,[13] and illegal trade in slaves, always significant, continued almost to the end of the nineteenth century. Its effect was to worsen the conditions of slave transport. Mortality ratios of eight ships captured by the English in 1830 were macabre: 72/258, 73/258, 47/300, 271/562, 680/983, 126/348, 39/144, and 216/422.[14] The phenomenal profit-taking by Cuban, Spanish, and

Table 3.1
Introduction of Slaves in Cuba*

Years	Havana	Totals	Years	Havana	Totals
1521-1762	—	60,000	1824	—	7,700
1763	1,700	—	1825	—	6,400
1764-89	24,875	33,409	1826	—	4,500
1790	2,534		1827	—	4,800
1791	8,498		1828	—	10,600
1792	8,528		1829	—	10,300
1793	3,777		1830	—	11,700
1794	4,164		1831	—	12,500
1795	5,832		1832	—	9,800
1796	5,711		1833	—	11,000
1797	4,452		1834	—	13,600
1798	2,001		1835	—	17,800
1799	4,919		1836	—	17,000
1800	4,145		1837	—	18,100
1801	1,659		1838	—	10,495
1802	13,832		1839	—	10,995
1803	9,671		1840	—	10,104
1804	8,923		1841	—	8,893
1805	4,999		1842	—	3,630
1806	4,395		1843	—	8,000
1807	2,565		1844	—	10,000
1808	1,607		1845	—	1,300
1809	1,162		1846	—	1,419
1810	6,672		1847	—	1,450
1811	6,349		1848	—	1,500
1812	6,081		1849	—	8,700
1813	4,770		1850	—	3,500
1814	4,321		1851	—	5,000
1815	9,111		1852	—	7,924
1816	17,737		1853	—	12,500
1817	25,841		1854	—	10,230
1818	19,902		1855-1857	—	9,000
1819	17,194		1858	—	16,000
1820	4,122		1859	—	12,000
1791-1820	—	281,794	1860	—	24,895
1821	—	10,000	1861	—	15,000
1822	—	4,500	1862	—	23,964
1823	—	2,000	1863-1873	—	60,000
			Total of slaves introduced		816,378

*From Juan Pérez de la Riva, "¿Cuántos africanos fueron traídos a Cuba?" *Economía y Desarrollo*, 1 (July-September 1970)3:141.

foreign slavers was buoyed by the falling price of slaves on the African coast caused by the English departure, and by the contrasting rise in the price of slaves in Cuba. The increased Cuban demand, naturally stimulated by threatened scarcity, was also supported by land reform, instigated by the Sociedad Económica, which generated new wealth by title grants for upwards of ten thousand Cuban landowners.[15] Romay's efforts to increase European immigration, I am sure, had the same effect.

Romay's Morality

Given the prevailing forces of the times, no special amount of greed, personal ambition, or moral weakness was needed to place the most talented and educated Cubans, like Romay, at the service of the evolving slavocracy. It was probably no easier for white Cubans to consider giving up slavery than it is today for North Americans to consider giving up their automobiles, war production, or economic growth. While Romay did not transcend the conditions of his social class or historical circumstance, he did express an advanced or at least elevated morality. Unlike many of his class brothers, Romay's style and sensibilities betrayed strong roots in a more stable past and in the self-righteously paternalistic and Catholic aristocracy. This background, and his strong ties to slavery, are expressed in his writings on the slave trade. Six years of experience innoculating *negros bozales* (recently arrived Africans) against smallpox acquainted Romay with the worst aspects of the slave trade. His revulsion prompted him, finally, in 1811, to protest the conditions of the trade. In an exposition directed to the Real Consulado, Romay explained that the horrible number of deaths had been caused by the overcrowding of small vessels; failure to provide bleeders, barbers, surgeons, or medicines of any kind; and the absence of adequate food, water, fresh air, and exercise for the slaves.

> It results thus, that from inobservation of these rules, or from miserable economizing and villany . . . men have died. . . . And on what occasion, . . . are these signs of most criminal ignorance and greed presented? . . . the conservation of agriculture of this island, the prosperity of some individuals, one would ask, is . . . preferable to the life of just one man? What are the much sung advantages that are acquired by these unfortunates, if they are hardly torn from their homes when they are entombed in the depths of the sea? Is it not better to live, although errant in the jungles, without permanent home, without law or religion, than to die from the arbitrary impunity of some men who do not recognize other rights than that of their own sordid interests?

Speaking of the slave ships that leave for Africa without adequate preparation, Romay commented bitterly:

> Neither sacks of coal nor bales [euphemisms of the slave trade] are
> what is going to be returned; they know very well that it is bound to
> be men, and although black and slave, they should be proportioned all
> the help required by humanity and ordered by our laws.

But Romay carefully defined his positon in favor of rationalized trade and
against *needless* suffering.

> I do not doubt that this aspect of my sensibility will bring me the
> hatred of those degraded souls that are suffocating in the most twisted
> wealth . . . It does not matter. They will know in the end that far from
> threatening their interest, I am procuring to augment [the number of
> slaves] with less risk and with responsibility. The cost of one thou-
> sand pesos, which soon will be how much the repairs of a surgeon and
> a chest of medicines will be worth on a round trip, will be successfully
> compensated, curing and conserving the health of only three blacks.
> And they [the slave traders] will be convinced of the rectitude of my
> intentions when they consider that I have a private motive to con-
> tribute to the augumented introduction of *negros bozales* in this port;
> thus if I tend to diminish it with the present motion, it is without
> doubt because I prefer the common good to my own utility and con-
> venience.[16]

Worsening Conditons of Slavery

But while slave imports jumped, the writings of Romay have nothing
to say about the conditions of the slave *in* Cuba. As the scale of sugar
production climbed, work became increasingly regimented, dehumanizing,
and impersonal. Beef and other foodstuffs were imported rather that ex-
ported as Cuba and her plantations lost their self-sufficiency in food and
even in fuel. Economic fluctuations brought "seasons of hunger," and
slaves lost not only their small gardens but most of their previously
respected rights. Sugar estates developed barracks (replacing the village-
like clusters of huts), infirmaries, and nurseries—conditions that were
reflected in the greater frequency of slave revolts on larger, more advanced
plantations.[17] The care of slaves also varied by their market value or
replacement cost. When prices were low, many slave owners followed an
explicit policy of working the slave to death as fast as possible, rather than
support women, children, and aged, incapacitated slaves.[18] Reflecting the
price of slaves and increased scale were the small hospital-infirmaries that
appeared as adjuncts to mills and barracks. Although having well-stocked
storerooms and sometimes the services of a Spanish physician,[19] the

infirmary was always regarded as an excuse for procrastination. This suspicion was reduced, however, by the frequent serious accidents caused by dangerous machinery in the mills, the well-known hazards of cutting cane, and, everywhere, the fatigue of overwork. An odd kind of safety equipment was the machete of the overseer, ready to cut off the erring hand caught in a roller. During harvest, slaves were made to work almost twenty hours daily on even the best run estates, kept awake by the whip of the overseer.[20]

The brutality of conditions is reflected by a variety of data. Suicide became such a problem that it was long the topic before the king's highest council.[21] While many abortions were apparently self-induced, pregnant women frequently lost their babies performing heavy work and suffering beatings up to the time of giving birth. Infants in turn suffered a mortality rate of one out of five.[22] In such context, epidemics, even of common colds, were quite serious, while smallpox, cholera, and diptheria left waves of death among the slave population.[23] Increasing regimentation, sexual anxieties, and short-sighted slave policies are suggested by shifting statistics of sexual composition: from 50,000 males and 40,000 females in 1792 to 125,000 and 25,000 respectively in 1817.[24] The lot of growing numbers of contract freedmen and Chinese, especially later in the nineteenth century, was even worse than that of slaves.

The desperate conditons of forced labor in Cuba were not helped by the climbing wealth and expanding production. At most, the slave received an ample diet in periods of good harvest and stable market. Chronic instabilities and anxieties were caused by continuously high interest rates and by a revolution in technology that was being capitalized on by agents of the slave trade, successful merchants, and foreign investors. Many estates were precariously cast in marginal positions that would hardly support a generous or far-sighted administration of slave labor. Moreover, the great boom in coffee production—which boasted superior labor conditions and almost paralleled sugar expansion in terms of slave labor employed after 1790—collapsed in the 1840s and left room for the complete hegemony of sugar.

WHITE POPULATION DEVELOPMENT

In 1811, the year of Romay's lament on the slave trade, the highly organized and far-reaching slave conspiracy of José Antonio Aponte caused alarm among slave owners, already made anxious by the increasing ratio of black over white population.[25] This national neurosis nourished a rather explicit racism in Romay's writings and led not to efforts to halt or decrease the slave trade, but to an effort to increase Catholic European immigration. As secretary of the White Population Development Board of the Sociedad Económica, Romay wrote an exposition in 1817, cosigned by the Havana Ayuntamiento (government council under the Spanish Constitution of 1812) and the Real Consulado, successfully urging that foreign Catholics be given liberties and incentives to settle in Cuba. His remarks, which should be considered in the context of its purpose, included the following argument:

> Although our agriculture is so precarious for lack of hands to develop it, only a necessity irreparable by other means obliges us to make use of a servant class so grievous as that of the blacks, for the great capital that is invested in them, for the little utility that their work produces as a consequence of their natural rudeness and indolence, and for the fear that is inspired in us by their increase over the number of whites.
>
> These fears are not as old as the slavery of blacks. More than two centuries we have lived tranquilly, although disgusted with their service.

The exposition, which failed to mention the 25,000 *negros bozales* imported in the same year, argued that the fear of slave rebellion was caused by abolitionism in England, France, and Spanish legislature; the proximity to Haiti; and the independence movements in Spanish America.

Protection of New Settlements

On the positive side, were it not for the racist and colonialist overtones, the Board on White Population could be regarded as a progressive economic and community planning agency. The board, also part of the Sociedad Económica, was instrumental in the planning and development of new towns and the recruitment of skilled immigrants to Cuba. Health conditions, which were a major consideration for many prospective immigrants, were studied carefully. Immigrants were urged to arrive in the winter months and discouraged from spending time in Havana, rife with yellow fever; temporary lodgings were provided a few miles inland, in the supposedly more healthy towns of Guanabacoa, Güines, and Guanajay. The new towns of Matanzas, Trinidad, Baracoa, Nipe, Cienfuegos, Guantánamo, Givar, Jagua, Mariel, and Nuevitas were developed, giving attention to distance from swamps and forests, thought to be the source of insalubrious atmospheric conditions. Houses were built to take the greatest advantage of summer breezes.[27] Whatever semblance of planning one could later find in mid-twentieth century cities was owed to early Spanish design and to the rationalized development in these first twenty-five years of the nineteenth century.

In the effort to secure the new populations, settlements of a certain size were sometimes provided the services of a salaried medical practitioner who was charged to administer free services to the poor.[28] Immigration itself included numbers of practitioners who were attracted by stories of Cuban wealth. In the period April through November 1818, for example, of 517 immigrant males, eleven were physicians and surgeons, the fourth largest category after farmers (320), carpenters (62) and brick layers (23). Six of the eleven were from France, and one each from Spain, England, the United States, Germany, and Italy.[29]

The efforts to obtain a larger white population and, where necessary, the purchase of lands for new settlement were supported by a tax of six pesos on every male *bozal* introduced in Cuban ports. Slavery, then, not only stimulated, but also financed the recruitment of white population. The efforts of white population development helped to stabilize the economy of sugar and, by a twist of economic dynamics, further stimulated the import of slaves.

SMALLPOX VACCINATION

Smallpox vaccination, which offered itself to the world at the beginning of the nineteenth century, tested the scientific and organizational abilities of medical and government authorities everywhere. If its acceptance and effective implementation seems to have been slow in Cuba, one might recall that the Royal London College of Physicians and Surgeons in Jenner's England failed for many years to endorse the lifesaving discovery. Smallpox continued to appear in London and Paris throughout the nineteenth century, and the victories of the Prussian over the French armies were influenced by the superior vaccination and sanitary program of the former. In comparison with other areas of Latin America, Cuba was early in developing a stable, if insufficient, program of smallpox vaccination.[30]

In Cuba, vaccination was fortunate to be championed by a man of Romay's stature. Following the success of Jenner's discovery as it was conclusively tested in England, parts of Europe and the United States, Romay offered through the pages of *Papel Periódico* a prize of 400 pesos to the person who successfully brought the vaccine to Cuba or discovered cowpox disease in Cuban herds. This awkward method was slow to bring results (slower at least than a fast Yankee slaver that could have been dispatched for such an important purpose to Philadelphia). One day, in February 1804, word was brought to Dr. Romay that a woman had just arrived from Puerto Rico, bringing with her a son and two servant girls who were vaccinated on the day of their departure from that island. Applying pus from the sores of these children and following directions offered by the Medical Board of Paris, Dr. Romay immediately vaccinated his own four children along with the children and young slaves of various luminaries of the Havana oligarchy and Amigos del País.[31]

The smallpox epidemic, which had been active in Havana since 1803 caused bedlam at the first public vaccination. Romay reported the event in the *Papel Periódico*:

> More than two hundred persons have been vaccinated by different professors from . . . the first children that were vaccinated on the twelfth and thirteenth of this month. But I doubt that the eruption will be verified in all that were vaccinated in my house in the afternoon of the twenty-first. The extraordinary gathering . . . and the pain with which many tried to be taken care of at the same time, deprived the physicians of operating in the light, of the action of their hands, and of the tranquility necessary to conduct a delicate, though simple, operation. I could do no more as a favor to the public than to generously present the three of my children who could be of use, in order that four professors could at the same time take from their delicate limbs the beneficent pus that preserves one from the most horrible death. This consideration overcame the just fear I had that they might be wounded in the midst of that disorder and confusion.[32]

Adding to the confusion, other practitioners and "intruders" elsewhere propagated the vaccine, often using ineffective or harmful methods. The first to seek innoculation were from already infected homes and erroneously attributed their consequent illness to the innoculation rather than to previous infection. Similar consequences followed the vaccination of those who were struck by other sickness common in Havana: whooping cough, acute diarrhea, measles, and yellow fever. Thus already in March, Romay began his long effort to discount in the press the many rumors which alleged the ineffectiveness or danger of vaccination. To this end, on March 23, Romay publicly innoculated his own children with live smallpox virus in order to dramatically demonstrate the effectiveness and safety of vaccination.[33]

The Central Vaccine Board

It was soon clear that a major problem would be the conservation of the vaccine virus itself. An uninterrupted innoculation had to be assured in a minimum number of children because cattle were not successfully used for this purpose. Romay proposed the establishment of a Central Vaccine Board and a plan for the vaccination of new slaves in the port, children in the orphanage, new babies in the palisade of the king's slaves, and every new baby within twelve days of birth. A room in the San Ambrosio military hospital was to be dedicated to the vaccination of new soldiers and immigrants, and virus material would be mailed under glass to practitioners in the interior. Finding approval of the plan, if not for its effective support, the Junta Central de Vacuna became another semigovernmental agency of the Sociedad Económica with Romay serving as its secretary until 1835. In this capacity he offered his services two days a week in the two Casas Capitulares (headquarters of ecclesiastic chapters) of Havana where vaccination was freely dispensed to all who presented themselves at times announced in the *Papel Periódico*.

The vaccine was distributed in a mostly unplanned fashion in the interior. Physicians, planters, and well-intentioned officials carried the vaccine, usually in the sores of children, to the towns, mills and haciendas of the interior. Some regions were fortunate to gain the services of practitioners who, like Romay, dedicated themselves to the maintenance and preparation of the vaccine. Romay himself carried the vaccine to one of the haciendas of his cousin and fellow member of the Sociedad Económica, the Conde de Casa Bayona. Here the surgeons and doctors from nearby towns and mills assembled to witness the operation and to carry the vaccine to their respective areas. The regions of Santa Clara, San Juan de los Remedios, and Sancti Spíritus, benefited from the work of an exemplary exponent of vaccination, the surgeon Juan Castellanos, who for years provided extensive service to these areas.

Resistance to Vaccination

Other areas, however were less fortunate: "*Bachiller* Joseph Bernal, physician of the city of Jaruco, sent a boy to carry the vaccine to his compatriots. With this, he tried to diffuse the vaccine in the nearby towns; but the ignorance and fanaticism became so opposed to his progress, that by the end of April he had vaccinated only two hundred nine subjects."[34] Similar problems were encountered in Santiago de Cuba, where the cowpox germs were introduced a month earlier than in Romay's Havana by a French physician from St. Thomas, Mr. Vignard, "lamenting that disconfidence and vulgar preoccupations obstructed their progress in a populous city that so much needed that help."[35] Even greater difficulties were encountered in the far western part of Cuba. One of the greatest obstacles was the curative orientation of traditional medicine, for it was popularly believed that vaccination was a *cure* for smallpox. Failing to grasp the concept of preventive medicine, parents securely waited to vaccinate their children until they showed symptoms of smallpox, only to be grieved by the prognosis of the innoculator.

Resistance to the vaccine was not, however, limited to the "vulgar." Many physicians and professors of medicine opposed vaccination, although official resistance was weakened or dissipated by the arrival, later in 1804, of a royal emissary charged with propagating the vaccine. A well-known Dr. Pachón declared the vaccine to be inauthentic and ineffective in an article in the *Papel Periódico* itself, arguing that Romay's treatment was without value because it did not cause a real case of smallpox, which was the object of older technique of innoculation.[36] Romay's answers are landmarks in the literature of public health polemic. With a careful logic and great zeal, Romay dissected the arguments of his opponents. The following quotation is noteworthy for its aggressiveness, at the end of a long and carefully reasoned article, "Refutation to Anti-Vaccinators:"

> I respect the prudence of some of our physicians, those who for a certain circumspection with which nobody may quarrel observe an inviolable silence on the vaccine, suspending for now their judgement. . . . How different is the conduct of other professors! Without calculating the prejudice that their premature vote can infer; without considering the authenticity and . . . number of proofs that support the preservative virtue of the vaccine; . . . They dissuade many unwary persons with disfigured facts or suppositions. *Infelices!* They have deprived the country of many useful citizens; they have covered with mourning the desolation of many families. The day will come in which, dissipated the clouds which darken their eyes, they will flee from the presence of those parents who they made shed bitter tears. Tormented by the remorse of their own conscience, made the object of public desecration and of popular scorn, . . . the anathemas of humanity will follow them to the tomb, the country will detest their memory, and the virtuous citizens will hang their names between Attila and Robespierre.[37]

In its first month the Central Vaccine Board published and made available to various practitioners a thousand copies of a technical guide to smallpox vaccination. In a genuine instance of popular health education, Romay published, by directive of the Central Vaccine Board, an "Instruction Directed to Mothers to Familiarize Them with Innoculation in Order that They Themselves Can Vaccinate their Children." The utility of these approaches was limited by the short reach of newspapers and by the low level of literacy,but their usefulness extended through the variety of practitioners who could be helped by the literature in their practice.

The Church

In addition to the formal and financial support of government, vaccination was supported by the highest official of the Church, the liberal bishop Dr. Díaz de Espada y Landa, director of the Sociedad Económica. On the arrival of the vaccine, he wrote to Romay, "As in my mansions are verified the general concurrence and reunion of all the children of the circumference, the healthy remedy can be prodigiously extended; being very agreeable the combination of coming to receive the Sacred Spirit by confirmation, they may return with those preservatives against a disease destructive in the temporal, and with this fortified for the spiritual career."[38] Touring his diocese in 1804, Díaz Espada was everywhere accompanied by a practitioner who vaccinated in his presence. Parish priests were instructed to urge innoculation at all baptisms and to announce on important holy days the time and place of public vaccination. The church was therefore the most important organization, aside from the slave market, which extended vaccination efforts beyond the pages of the *Papel* and to ordinary people. Of all methods, pastoral announcements seem to have been the most important in certain cities of the interior. But in 1805, seeing the meager fruits of their efforts thus far, the Vaccine Board persuaded the bishop to again require that parents be informed of the method and benefit of innoculation. Priests were charged to record, not only the names of the parents, but their addresses as well, in order that personnel of the Vaccine Board, whenever they found themselves without someone to receive the vaccine, could solicit subjects from among the newborn and their families. But even these measures were as limited as the narrow extention of the church of Cuba to principal towns and cities. At no time did the vaccination of the newborn exceed one-third of the registerd baptisms, more than 300 per month after 1805 in Havana.[39]

The small but growing number of primary schools provided another important organization for the promotion of the new vaccine, and Romay's parallel participation in the Sociedad's efforts in public education probably facilitated the use of these new institutions for smallpox vaccination. Vaccination of school children was already successful before it became mandatory in 1817, and the health record of the young scholars became a strong argument in favor of Romay's public health propaganda.[40].

In 1805, in Santa María del Rosario, the constant efforts of physician José Govín were institutionalized at his request in the form of a Junta Subalterna de Vacuna. Seeing the logic of this method, the central board eventually established, through the respective regional deputations of the Sociedad, other Subalternate Boards in Trinidad, Camagüey, and Santiago de Cuba. In Santiago, the work was financed by a tax of two pesos per slave introduced in that port. These methods were supplemented and assisted by the frequent dispatching of vaccine to towns, mills and haciendas of the interior, usually upon the outbreak of the disease.

Mixed Success

The overall success of the work of the vaccine boards was constantly frustrated and often the main objective was reduced to the preservation of the vaccine virus. Once, for example, in 1805, the vaccine, which had been innoculated in only one person, was feared lost when the innoculation sores were scratched and the transmitability of the vaccine destroyed. But by chance the slave's sores had been used to vaccinate other children in the home and thus the continuity of vaccine was saved in Cuba.

Joseph Bernal, Juan Castellanos, José Govín and others who propagated the vaccine in the interior should be regarded as the precursors of the new public health physician. Largely unrecorded in the history of their time, they served the needs of their communities with dedication for many years. Unfortunately, in most areas the initial efforts were abandoned and most rural areas were continually without access to vaccination. For lack of government support and organization the good works of many individuals could not become a genuine public health service.

Sadly, the greatest popular incentive continued to be the threat posed by sporadic cases of the disease and recurrent epidemic. Eight hundred children were buried in the general cemetery in 1803, a great year of epidemic. But 1804, the year in which vaccination began, produced Romay's most frequently cited statistic. Calculating to preserve the great fear of smallpox, he forever recalled the 800 victims of smallpox who in 1804 were entombed "in just one church." Epidemic returned in 1812 to Puerto Príncipe, Bayamo, and other cities of the interior and went unchecked throughout the entire year. It struck again in 1816 and extended to Havana in 1817. The epidemic returned to Trinidad, Sancti Spíritus and Santa Clara in 1828, continuing in 1829 even in Havana.[41]

Although Romay failed to achieve the goal of smallpox eradication, the disease was partially contained. Highly valued high risk populations were preserved—new slaves, immigrants, and students. Privileged groups were protected—the oligarchy and some readers of the Papel Periódico, as well as their slaves and servants. Vaccination campaigns against epidemic targets were helpful. Altogether, smallpox vaccination saved many lives and limited the velocity, scope, and frequency of smallpox contagion. The reappearance of smallpox through the remainder of the nineteenth century is testimony to inadequate organizational forms and insufficient efforts directed toward the common people, especially in rural Cuba.

Romay's judgement, in 1819, although perhaps beyond criticism in his time, reveals the root of failure in an elitist, voluntaristic, top-down approach to public health:

> [The constant propagation of smallpox] should not be imputed to a lack of zeal and vigilence in the government for the public health, nor to ommission of the central board in charge of propagating the vaccine. Its medical members attend without fail on Wednesdays and Saturdays at the Casas Capitulares to innoculate or supply their virus under glass to *whomever asks* [my emphasis]. Another professor dispenses with the same generosity . . . in the parish of Nuestra Señora de Guadalupe. In the neighborhoods of Jesús María, Jesús del Monte,

and in different towns, there also reside practitioners of accredited instruction and humanity.[42]

The methodology assumed a cultural level and an access to information
that was nonexistent or limited to certain sectors of the population. In addition to making services available, direct outreach and mild coercion was
necessary. The desparation of the elitist method is suggested by Romay's at
least half serious conclusion:

> If smallpox were to entirely disappear, the most incontestable argu-
> ment would be lacking for the efficacy of its preservative, and losing
> the horror and even the idea of that disease, it could not be procured to
> prevent it. It is thus necessary for the conservation of the vaccine
> virus that there be some people so stupid or negligent . . . in order that
> the smallpox contagion will gloat itself on these, leaving untouched
> the vaccinated and the beneficient fluid may be perpetuated, recom-
> mending itself with repeated counterproofs.[43]

Under the arrogance of a protected and self-satisfied oligarchy, the ends of
public health were callously displaced by their means.

The decline of slave imports and the end of their tax revenue after
1821 (when the trade became illegal), the imposition of a more conservative
and dictatorial Spanish government in 1823, and increased government
graft (as Creole exclusion from offices was strengthened) hastened the
financial crisis, collapse, and inactivity of the Subalternate Boards of the
interior.[44] Even in Santiago, an effort had to be made to reestablish their
presence to face the epidemics of 1827 and 1828. The epidemics of these
years and the disruption they caused seem to have demonstrated to Romay
that smallpox vaccination could only be successful if it was directed to the
broadest public health objective. He was forced to admit the inefficacy of
newspaper pronouncements and rudimentary availability. The need for a
more coercive approach, which was never in fact effected except in the foci
of epidemics, was clear to Romay in 1827 when he reported, "Not doubted
today that the innoculation of the vaccine is as simple as it is beneficial,
nobody refuses it when it is dealt to him in his own house."[45] But Romay
lacked the means or the imagination to effect the neighborhood approach
suggested by his own observation. Without an organized medical class,
supportive popular organizations, or adequate finance, the most Romay
could do was to recognize and promote a frail principle of paternalistic
coercion. In areas of epidemic, police orders called upon citizens to appear
with their children for vaccination, on pain of a fine of ten *ducados*. This
successful method was supplemented by another rather morbid form of
coercion: quarantine camps were built outside of towns, forcing the dis-
eased into deliberately inadequate facilities, without provision for different

sexes, calculated to add horror to disease and urgency to vaccination.[46] These measures were justified by principles which, fortunately, have since been more appropriately implemented: "The conservation of the vaccine is not a business of private interest, but a public utility and convenience."[47]

REFORM IN MEDICAL EDUCATION

The thrust of Romay's work in medical education was to secularize medicine. First, medicine was removed from a hierarchy of medical priesthood and sacred texts; second, medicine and health became subjects to analyze in ways common to such prosaic matters as agriculture and economics; and, third, medicine became something that could be learned and applied by ordinary men, using ordinary abilities, without the use of mysterious words, manners, or secret potents. These changes were of course incomplete and did not immediately produce great medicine. Romay's own medicine was a combination of crude epidemiology, naive clinical induction, rationalist speculation and attempted application of foreign medical developments, of which there were few. The shortcomings of Romay's revolution in medicine were not unique to him or to Cuba; the central dilemma of eighteenth century medicine lay in its slowness to develop practical applications for its great discoveries in physiology and chemistry. While much of old medical lore had been decisively discredited, it was not yet clear what the new science would prescribe for its patients.[48].

But the slowness of scientific method to produce practical results should not belittle the importance of having introduced a new frame of mind. The unenlightened eighteenth-century university, founded by Dominicans, was run like an isolated, austere monastery. At the turn of the century it still offered a course on "mathematics and their meaning for our King and God." Even in 1816, when Romay argued for the establishment in the military hospital of a new school of practical anatomy and clinical medicine, he could say:

> The physiology and pathology which is taught in the classrooms of this University . . . still render reason to fragments, oppressed and foggy, not only with frivolous questions . . . , but also with errors that are very prejudicial to conservation of health. They still teach that the four elements are the constitutive principles of all beings; that the sanguification and segregation of the other three humors which they call primary, are performed in the liver; that all illnesses are similar, organic and common; that the similarities are called *intemperies*, etc. But what could be the theory of Lazaro Riviero [the texts still used in the University], having written in the sixteenth century? When

Harvey had not discovered the circulation of the blood, nor had Haller sketched the first lines of physiology, nor Ludwig conceived his pathology, nor Bichar applied anatomy in physiology and medicine.[49]

Systematic Teaching in Hospitals

The dismal state of medical education at the time of Romay's writing is further expressed by Romay's desperation at not finding a single physician or professor in Cuba who had studied practical clinical medicine in Europe and who could thus guide the development of the new program. The new program of studies had to be improvised from what could be read about the hospital-schools of Europe and by self-education in the new sciences. The program that was established in the military hospital sounds familiar today: history taking, hospital rounds with the professor, case presentation by students and professors, record keeping and follow-up review of patients.[50] There would be no theory, said Romay, with his characteristic naiveté, and the only texts would be "the cadaver, the patient, and the effects they can produce on our own sensory organs." These observations, he would add, should then be compared with those reported in the new medical literature of Europe. Record keeping under Romay's direction gave great attention to atmospheric temperature and weather conditions, which were not altogether irrelevant to tropical health, and also, to leave no stone unturned, the rigor of observation included the "state of meteors." Confronted by a battle among several systems and schools of thought, Romay preached a dogma of eclecticism. In the formal inauguration of clinical courses in San Ambrosio, Romay rather poetically exhorted his students, "As the bee extracts from flowers the purest nectar to convert it into a useful and very sweet honey, so also you shall take from each school the doctrines most in conformity to strict reason, to repeated and analyzed facts, to principles generally admitted, in order to form a collective system, the surest one in the difficult science of curing."[51]

Gaining a victory over the reactionary university, the Protomedicato was influenced to consider training in practical anatomy and clinical medicine as prerequisites for licensure in medicine. A *bachillerato* in medicine (a degree of secondary education, awarded in Romay's time by the university after three years of study) was prerequisite for the hospital programs; other university students took the clinical courses after earning their licenciate degree. Two separate programs existed. The graduates of San Ambrosio gained no formal titles but they could be licensed to practice medicine as physicians and surgeons; the graduates of the university could gain a formal title (licenciate) which effectively permitted the student to practice medicine, but he could not be licensed by the Protomedicato without completing courses in San Ambrosio. The two medicines coexisted. Although there is nothing in the literature against scholasticism approaching the antagonism of Romay's attack on the antivaccinators, there was significant strain between the two schools.

The Sociedad Económica financed part of the new hospital program and also professorships in the university proper. Through this power certain aspects of teaching were influenced. The teaching of anatomy by the use of wax figures was largely discontinued in favor of cadavar dissection and clinical observation, and scholarships were awarded for scientific study in Europe. In 1823, with the overthrow of the liberal Spanish constitution of 1812 and the suppression of a constitutionalist conspiracy in Cuba, the new captain general ordered the termination of university courses in constitutional philosophy given by the liberal abolitionist, Father Félix Varela. While Varela fled into exile, the one thousand pesos per year that were saved by the suppression of his courses were diverted, upon Romay's benign recommendation, to a professor of descriptive anatomy, operations, and art of child delivery.[52] In 1827, a school for midwives was also established in the women's hospital, San Francisco de Paula.

Whatever the criticism or merit of medical education, it did not affect many students. There were some ten students in the classes of the medical school at the turn of the century,[53] and not more than thirty students in the courses of San Ambrosio by 1825. Thus increasing medical immigration was especially significant for Cuba and lesser practitioners continued to predominate in the provision of most medical care.

In 1834, the institution of the Protomedicato was replaced by a Royal Governing Board of Medicine and Surgery. When Romay was named president of this board, the security of the new hospital courses and their eventual incorporation in university reform was assured. The security of Romay's orientation was also assured by Romay's own good health, for the oldest graduate of each school automatically became dean of that faculty. Thus, by 1842, when university reform was finally promulgated and the university was officially secularized, Romay at age 78 was dean not only of the medical school (after 1833), but of the school of philosophy as well. Considering that he was also the director of the Sociedad Económica, he was clearly in the odd position—after working to discredit the sacred texts—of having become the high priest of Cuban medicine.

PHARMACEUTICAL REGULATIONS

Aside from licensure of physicians and surgeons, and the pompous proclamation of the Hippocratic Oath, the Royal Governing Board probably exerted little governance over the practical activities of most practitioners. Rising prosperity and growing numbers of practitioners seems in the same period to have led to a certain commercial spirit, especially among everyday practitioners.

The petty entrepreneurial phenomenon in health is reflected in the 1843 Governing Board's "Report and Regulation on Secret and New Medicines."[54] This report is probably one of the first serious attempts to regulate everyday medical practice. The traffic in new and secret potions had reached alarming dimensions and was founded on "the greed of some men and the credulity of the ignorant and vulgar." A scientific sounding or mysterious label, careful and detailed instructions, and certification by one or many real or imaginary eminent practitioners was the familiar form. Practitioners were tempted, the report continues, to seek "immoderate" wealth and the public was swindled as it inclined toward novelty, secrets, and mystery. Accidents and some alleged deaths resulted while the "infestation of the population with inert, weak, or dangerous remedies" caused people to forget tried and successful remedies, thus contributing to the eclipse of "true medicine." The traffic induced some physicians to dedicate themselves wholly to the prescription or concoction of these secret potions. And these, even when really new, seldom enriched the stock of medicines, for they at best duplicated the effects of existing remedies. The report concluded that the flood of new remedies made impossible the control and prevention of fraudulent imitations. The ensuing regulation banned new and secret medicines not approved by the Inspección de Estudios, an office under the Governing Board, reserving the submission of new medicines to professors of medicine and surgery. "Prejudicial" medicines were not to be allowed and others were to be marked either "equivalent to medicines already known" or "more effective that those already known." Moreover, the Inspección would determine the *price* of approved medicines.

The attempted regulation indicates the progress of legitimate practitioners that was necessary for regulation to be remotely realistic. At the same time the underlying message of the report is clear: the first medical revolution, while it combated obscurantism in the academy, had little effect on the obscurantism of the medical practice which affected the largest number of Cubans. In fact, economic expansion increased the numbers and wealth of every kind of practitioner and every kind of practice.

HOSPITALS

The unpardonable spirit of commerce seems to have also made its way into hospital care. Although no private hospitals were formed or known by that classification, there were houses that advertised care for the sick. Especially in times of epidemic, these houses sprang up all over the city. Their chief advertisement was the unpopular reputation of regular hospital services and their frequently insufficient capacity. A long tradition existed for the hospitals themselves to supplement their facilities with rented houses. By 1827 the increasing frequency and scope of yellow fever epidemic had given impetus to the establishment of private houses, even on the principal streets, which specialized in the treatment of the disease. It was the growth of these socially offensive establishments that caused Romay—who did not then believe, as he had in 1793, that yellow fever was contagious—to accept a plan for the quarantine of yellow fever victims in a quarantine camp outside the city:

> [The private homes for the sick] are not only contrary to health policy, because, multiplying the houses of corruption, the atmosphere that we breathe is more and more altered; but also because they sensibly offend the neighbors with the lament and complaining of the sick and dying and with the sight of cadavers that are frequently extracted; and besides, because the unhappy ones who prefer these houses to the public hospitals are not treated with the humanity and compassion that their sufferings call for; there is speculation [in their sufferings] . . . and they become the object of the most criminal profit.[55]

Actually these establishments, hardly mentioned in Cuban hospital history, are the real precursors of the *quintas de salud* or *clínicas de salud* which later developed. The most respectable early form was the dedication of nearby country homes of the rich (some of wealthy physicians) to the victims of epidemic. *Quinta*, which means "country house," later became almost synonomous with *clínica* and *casa de salud*. The quarantine regulations and the constant presence of susceptable travelers and new immigrants provided incentive for profitable conversion of *quintas* to small private infirmaries or hospitals.

Among the most reputable and prestigious of these early private hospitals was one founded in 1821 by Carlos Belot Lorent, a young Frenchman graduated from the University of Paris. The clinic was located in Regla, a short ferry trip from Havana and easily accessible to all vessels anchored in the bay of Havana. Belot's bold entrance to the hospital business was facilitated by exceptional qualifications as a clinician and strategic social connections. When he was absent from the clinic, his first replacement was Protophysician of Havana, Don Lorenzo Hernández (Romay's early teacher). Most of Belot's hospitalized patients from 1821 to 1824 were foreign Protestants. Owing to the fact that the local priest forbade their burial in his cemetery, Belot also acquired land and provided interment services. High sanitary standards, discipline, and general success made the clinic a model for others.[56] Notably, this and other small private hospitals (and even the large mutualist hospitals which come later) were not referred to as hospitals but rather as *casas de salud, quintas,* or *clínicas.*

The hospitals described in Romay's writings added more complex recordkeeping, formal teaching functions, and greater size. San Francisco de Paula was completely renovated—with funds derived from upper class charity— and expanded from 1777 to 1799. It had positions for physician, surgeon, bleeder, pharmacist, steward, cook, mother, three nurses or female attendants, and the distinguished Ladies of the City who alternated weeks to present lunch and supper and to serve as nurses, leaving copious sums in the little alms boxes of the House.[57] San Francisco de Paula also housed the female mentally ill whenever there was insufficient room in the women's house of correction. But this practice was discontinued when the unfortunate women were sent to share with senile and aged slaves a wing of the new poorhouse, the Casa de Beneficencia.

It was in San Francisco de Paula that Cuba's first formally trained female physician was imprisoned. Enriqueta Faber y Caven, graduate of the University of Paris and a heroic but unknown figure in women's history, immigrated to Cuba disguised as a man in 1821. After practicing three years in the small eastern town of Bayamo and serving as the local agent of the Protomedicato, her sex was discovered and she was charged with perjury and falsification of public documents. Fortunately, she was defended by a dedicated and influential jurist, Don Manuel Lorenzo de Vidaurre, who resigned his judgeship with the Real Audiencia de Príncipe to conduct her defense. Faber was also defended by the aging liberal Bishop Espada Landa. The crime, said her defense, was not hers but that of the society which forced her, the widow of a French army surgeon, to don male attire in order to survive and practice the healing profession. After twice escaping from San Francisco de Paula, Enriqueta Faber was exiled from all Spanish territory. Arriving in New Orleans, she joined the Sisters of Charity and eventually became an officer of high rank and esteem in the sisterhood. Her life, which is barely noted in this paragraph or in any other historical account known to me, deserves its own book. But this brief attention serves to illustrate the continuing imprisonment and oppression of women in the nineteenth century.[58]

The male insane, in this progressive era, were removed from the jail to the leprosarium, the Hospital de San Lázaro, next to the new cemetery. Here they stayed until the Hospital de San Dionisio, next to San Lázaro, was completed by Bishop Díaz Espada for the male insane in 1828. Neither of these establishments enjoyed regular attention by physicians.[59] Romay considered the leprosarium to be one of the "infectious" places and ordered that the quarantine of fever victims should be as distant as possible from San Lázaro and from the cemetery.

The cemetery itself was also the result of sanitary efforts by Romay and Bishop Díaz Espada, after whom the cemetery was named, to end the practice of burial in the church vaults. From 1802 to 1804, about two thousand three hundred were buried in the church vaults. This peculiar overpopulation caused the tombs to be opened every year to gather skeletons and add new bodies at a faster rate than usually recommended, and "the churches were infested with the fetid odour they exhaled." Again, the spirit of profit was involved. "The superstition of the faithful and the greed of the ecclesiastics have profaned the temples," Romay commented.[60]

Meanwhile, in the interior, there was hospital construction in Matanzas, Remedios, Sancti Spíritus, and Trinidad. In Puerto Prícinipe the general hospital expanded and added more facilities for military patients in 1827, the women's hospital was rebuilt in 1825, and in 1827 the leprosarium was also reconstructed. Santiago de Cuba added a women's hospital in 1825, the gift of a Don Emilio Prado. After the slave conspiracies and a thwarted nationalist-constitutionalist rising in 1823, the Spanish dictatorship established military infirmaries in several new inland towns.[61]

The religious mission of the hospital was mildly challenged in this period and the administration of the general hospital of Havana was taken from the holy friars and placed in the hands of municipal officials.[62] Romay wrote on the building of hospitals: "This does not require the recommendation of religion. Nature itself energetically asks that these monuments to humanity be established. Plato orders it in his laws, the Incas of Peru execute it, and the Muslims observe it." But the financial mechanism to carry out Plato's law also needed philosophical interpretation: "Providence . . . has conceded to some what to others has been denied, in order that the first exercise charity and the second patience: the former give away the superfluous and the latter receive the necessary. Naturally, these riches that I possess should not be enjoyed by me alone, but should be divided with the unfortunate and alleviate their pains."[63]

The most impressive manifestation of these principles was the Casa de Beneficencia, often admired for its solid architecture. A monument to humanity and also to its liberal benefactors, the construction of the Casa de Beneficencia marked an advance in the curative function and concept of the hospital, for it responsibly removed the problems of convalescence, infirmity, and destitution to a specialized institution. An improvement over the Arcos de Belén, the new house of charity inspired Romay to poetry. His poem "A la Casa De Beneficencia, En el Día de Sus Exámenes" contained these interesting verses:

> Live tranquilly, innocent souls,
> In this fortress of charity,
> She has inspired useful resources
> For you to share.

Raise to heavens your pure hands
Direct thankful voices, innocents
For the pious liberal souls
That favor you.[64]

The focus on Romay, I hope, has not seriously distorted his real historical role. A medical revolution and smallpox vaccination would certainly have followed European influences sooner or later. Moreover, the class of which Romay was part was determined to effect such changes. Other medical contemporaries of Romay would no doubt offer illuminating biographies, but others, especially the lower practitioners, left few records of their work. Social position, professional work, and official role caused Romay to leave behind a wealth of data on his interaction with the environment of his day. Neither saint nor devil, Romay reveals the moral, political, and intellectual contradictions of his time. His note of aristocratic and Hippocratic self-righteousness, tainted by the pragmatism of economic development and slavery, accurately reflects the social extraction and social position of the highest medical class. Romay was not a man to transcend his social circumstance, nor could he have been and preserved his social position. But he forever labored to achieve consistency between constructive public service and the elements of a moral order.

NOTES

1. If not wealthy, at least influential. The new suburban growth gave rise to many complaints from neighbors about the unsanitary and overcrowded hospital, causing the *regidores* of the city to plan a new location. See del Pino y de la Vega, p. 32.

2. This was also a sign of wealth; substantial sums were required to enter a monastic house and the houses, or chapters, had greatly enriched themselves over several generations. There were only around 150 monks and of these, most were of upper class background. See, for example, Thomas, p. 40.

3. See notes in Thomas, p. 5 and p. 53.

4. Ibid., p. 32.

5. José López Sánchez, *Tomás Romay and the Origins of Science in Cuba*, translated by Mary Todd Haessler (Havana: Book Institute, 1967), p. 20. His brothers-in-law were Rafael (a jurist and advisor to the Cabildo, the Royal Consulate, and the Royal Merchantile Tribunal) and Friar Juan ("religious orator and panegirist of Luis de las Casas", who was the Captain-General of Cuba).

6. Thomas, p. 62.

7. Ibid., p. 72.

8. See table of slave imports in "Romay and Slavery."

9. See Leuchsenring, p. 54 and López Sánchez, pp. 33-40.

10. López Sánchez, p. 211.

11. Thomas, p. 80.

12. Thomas, p. 84. This process is the key to the composition of the higher

social classes in nineteenth century Cuba: ". . . the slave trade, now as at the beginning in the 1760's, often provided not only the labour for the advancement of this industry but the capital as well; and the merchant, slaver or not, who also had a plantation was in a sense the only free planter."

13. This thesis is convincingly argued by Eric Williams, *Capitalism and Slavery* (New York: Russell and Russell, 1961).

14. Thomas, p. 163.

15. Ibid., p. 95.

16. Tomás Romay y Chacón, *Obras completas* 2 vols., compiled with an introduction by José López Sánchez, (Havana: Museo Histórico de las Ciencias Médicas "Carlos J. Finlay," 1965), vol. 1, p. 247.

17. Thomas, p. 63, especially p. 176.

18. For a confession of a progressive planter, see Knight, pp. 75-76.

19. Thomas, p. 179.

20. See Ibid., pp. 173-79 and Knight, p. 73 for descriptions of work conditions.

21. In the period 1847-55; see Knight, p. 78.

22. Thomas, p. 171.

23. 1833-34 epidemics of cholera brought an "integrated" Cuban death toll to more than 30,000; and together with smallpox the same disease again took a large toll of the slave population in 1850-1852. José A. Martínez-Fortún y Foyo, "Epidemiología (síntesis cronológica)," *Cuadernos de Historia Sanitaria, no. 5,* (Havana: Ministerio de Salubridad y Asistencia Social, 1952), pp. 31-32.

24. For conventional figures on slave population, 1774-1861, see Thomas, p. 169.

25. The ratio of black and mulatto to white flipped between 1792-1840 from 40%:60% to 60%:40%. (Ibid., p. 169.)

26. Romay, vol. 2, p. 141.

27. For a treatment of efforts to secure healthful conditions for new immigrants, see Romay, vol. 2, pp. 144-51.

28. Ibid., p. 170.

29. Ibid., p. 151.

30. See various discussions in Moll, especially pp. 234-35.

31. The illustrious figures were: Pedro Montalvo, Juan de Zazas, María Luisa Echeverría, Micaela Sánchez, Juan Manuel O'Farrill, Mariana O'Farrill, María Bustamente, Ignacio Pedroso, Juan Tomás de Juaregui, and Martín de Aróstegui. (Romay, vol. 1, p. 165.)

32. Ibid., pp. 167-68.

33. Ibid., p. 177.

34. Ibid., p. 205.

35. Ibid., p. 206. But for obvious reasons, Romay and not Mr. Vignard is remembered for having introduced smallpox vaccination to Cuba.

36. A highly controversial and rather widely practiced method of immunization employed small quantities of material from real smallpox sores in order to cause a mild case of the disease.

37. Ibid., p. 182.

38. Cited in Romay, p. 205.

39. Ibid., p. 216.

40. Actually, the orphans in the Casa de Beneficencia were the best advertisement, while negligence in the schools caused Romay to propose in 1817 a rigidly compulsory program for all students. Ibid., p. 279.

41. Ibid., pp. 229, 284, and 304.

42. Romay, vol. 1, p. 238.

43. Ibid., p. 223.

44. Ibid., p. 296.

45. Ibid., p. 287.

46. Ibid., p. 298.

47. Ibid.

48. The medical work of the eighteenth century lay the basis for the nineteenth century medical progress. See: Lester S. King, *The Medical World of the Eighteenth Century* (Chicago: U. of Chicago Press, 1958).

49. Romay, vol. 1, pp. 37-38.

50. Ibid., pp. 36-40.

51. Ibid., pp. 53-54.

52. Ibid., p. 44. Father Félix Varela was the first to teach logic and the first to lecture in the vernacular in the Cuban university.

53. Martínez Fortún y Foyo, *Apuntes*, p. 13.

54. Romay, vol. 1, pp. 57-61.

55. Ibid., p. 97.

56. In its first years, from August 1821 to September 1824, the clinic hospitalized 535 patients, of whom 120 died. The 535 patients included 185 Frenchmen, 116 Germans and Danes, 75 English, 76 North Americans, 59 Dutch, 21 Swiss, and 3 Spanish. Most of the deaths were from yellow fever. See Eduardo Gómez Luaces, "Regla: Su aporte a la medicina cubana en el siglo XIX," *Cuadernos de Historia de Salud Pública, no. 57*, (Havana: Ministerio de Salud Pública, 1973), pp. 29-33, 57-59.

57. Ibid., p. 116.

58. de Laura, pp. 97-99, and Roig de Leuchsenring, pp. 23-24.

59. del Pino y de la Vega, p. 41.

60. Romay, vol. 1, p. 141.

61. del Pino y de la Vega, pp. 43-46.

62. Ibid., p. 33.

63. Romay, vol. 1, p. 115.

64. Romay, vol. 2, pp. 249-51.

4
The Second
Medical Revolution,
1898-1922

CARLOS J. FINLAY

The dateposts of the second medical revolution are the first U.S. intervention of 1898 and the founding of the Federation of University Students in 1922. The stability and rising prosperity ensuing after the end of warfare in 1898 boosted government work in public health and provided a field for a revolution in medical practice based on international medical advances of the previous forty years. The founding of the Federation of University Students, within the university reform movement, is an event which at once marks the failings of the first two decades of independence and sounds the emergence of a new generation of activism for institutional reform that belongs to the following revolutionary period.

The central figure of the second medical revolution in Cuban history is Cuba's most famous physician, Carlos J. Finlay. Known for the discovery of the transmission of yellow fever by the mosquito, it is more appropriate, if not more precise, to remember Finlay as a great champion of scientific method and unity between social and clinical medicine. In an era of pseudoscientific patriarchs, governmental obstructions, and narrow clinical preoccupations, Finlay's life presents a story of battles on all fronts of medicine. Finlay was more completely a physician than Romay, while medical science emerged from a category under encyclopedism into an increasingly specialized and effective scientific vocation. Unlike Romay, Finlay was unattached to positions of political, economic, social, or academic power until the very end of his medical career. Thus the biography of Finlay provides less direct information on the social context of medicine, and it is necessary to preface biographical material with a dis-

69

cussion of social, economic, and medical institutional environments. The victories and decline of the second medical revolution are told in the passage from U.S. military rule to the early republic.

MEDICAL SYNOPSIS

The years from 1823 to 1860 were years of affluent inertia within the institutions and processes described in the first revolutionary period. The high patriarchy of Cuban medicine was passed from Romay to his bedside physician, Nicolás Gutiérrez, who, in 1861, became the founding president of the Cuban Academy of Medical, Physical, and Natural Sciences. Study abroad, preferably in France, became an established pattern for the Creole bourgeoisie and other young men of "good" family. This direction was argued with a mix of Cuban institutional inferiority, cosmopolitan decadence, prosperity, and genuine pursuit of intellectual excellence. Conflict between Spanish and Creole, heightened under Captain-General Tacón after 1833, diverted more privileged youth away from public careers and into less sensitive professions such as medicine and, increasingly, dentistry.

Although formally secularized in 1842 and influenced by Romay's rather basic reforms, the University of Havana was hardly progressive or technically advanced by the standards of the time. The most advanced medical practice was found among immigrant physicians and Cubans who studied abroad. The vanguard of Cuban science had shifted, not from the Sociedad Económica to the university, but to the new academy. Even this institution proved to be rather conservative, and probably resembled too closely the vainglorious university.

The lethargy of the university was deeply rooted in two pervasive colonial traditions: first, that public offices had come to be regarded as the personal property of their occupants and, second, that older office holders were automatically granted greater prestige and liberties. Everywhere, then, were the patterns of paternalism and patriarchy. The old professors did not relinquish their hold on positions until they died, assigning their functions to favorite substitutes, who in turn stood in the shadow of the great old man until a moment of opportunity arose. At such a moment, the protegé received the support of the old patriarch and was favored over other unprotected young men. The paradigm of this pattern was evidenced when the younger man not only inherited the position left vacant by the death or retirement of his protector, but also married the protector's daughter.

The patriarchs of the medical school were blessed, like Romay, with longevity. Thus, there was only one professor of surgery for almost the whole of the nineteenth century, Fernando González del Valle.[1] Receiving his ring and sword[2] from Romay, F. González del Valle left his professorship only when he died in 1881. Another exemplary figure of the nineteenth century university was Juan M. Bustamente. Long the substitute for his predecessor in anatomy and dissection, he acquired the position of his protector[3] in 1856 and held it until dying of tuberculosis in 1882, one year after replacing Fernando González del Valle as rector of the university. He was succeeded by his own substitute, José L. Yarini. Bustamente had raced through medical training to his position in the university. Beginning medical courses in 1842, he was assisting in dissections in 1843 and was a salaried dissecting assistant in 1844,[4] before he earned his bachillerato after the required six years in 1848. The questions asked in his examination were innocuous. Of three questions, one was "Can one practice surgery without knowing surgical anatomy?"[5] In less than two years after this tedious examination, Bustamente won his licenciate and doctorate degrees. When he submitted himself to the oral competition for the vacated professorship in 1856 only one other person was qualified to apply, Ramón Zambrana, whose brother Antonio happened to be rector of the university. To quiet a controversy over conflicting interests, the bishop of Havana quietly appointed Ramón to the directorship of the San Ambrosio military hospital (which had moved after 1827 to occupy the buildings of the defunct Royal Tobacco Factory). Bustamente's legacy, like that of others in the university was more than spiritual, although his bibliography seems to number no more than two articles. His first daughter married José Pulido Pagés, who at that time gained a professorship in the medical school. One son, Antonio (1865-1951), became professor of international law; a younger son, Alberto (1868-1950), became professor of obstetrics.[6]

Martyrdom of Eight Medical Students

The functions of the medical school were long centered around the old Hospicio de San Isidro, while the teaching of anatomy and dissection was variously located in San Ambrosio and in San Juan de Dios, with an occasional dissection of a female cadaver performed in the women's hospital, San Francisco de Paula. In 1870 some of the teaching functions, including anatomy and dissection were moved, with questionable wisdom, to the former San Dionisio hospital for mental patients that had been situated since 1826 next to the leprosarium on the edge of the Espada General Cemetery. As the first War for Independence (1868-1878) raged across Cuba, it was here in 1871 that an angry mob of Spanish Voluntarios[7] seized some thirty-eight first year medical students who were accused (falsely, it seems) of having scratched the new tomb of a martyred leader of the Voluntarios. Eight students were executed; thirty were sentenced to long prison terms.[8]

Modest university reform after 1880 in the interwar years, from 1879 to 1894, led to the dean of each school being elected by its cloister of professors from among the older one-half of its members, while the rector continued to be appointed by the captain-general. The first three years of secondary education (which terminated with the degree of *bachiller*) were finally separated from the university in an Institute of Secondary Instruction.

Colegio Médico Cubano

The interwar years brought a surge of professional medical activity outside of the university. Enríquez Núñez led his colleagues in the creation of the Colegio Médico Cubano, local associations of physicians devoted to cultural and scientific meetings, but with no real power over practitioners or power to defend their interests. In 1893, student associations were being formed and, influenced by Spanish syndicalism, a short lived dental union was formed.[9]. The first genuine medical journal was Santos Fernández's *Crónica Médico Quirúrgica*, supported by the Havana Society for Clinical Studies. In 1887, Santos Fernández also inaugurated the Quinta de Toga, Cuba's first medical laboratory, which soon produced antirabies serum and, in 1899, horse-derived serum against diptheria. Claudio Delgado installed the first stove contraption for sterilization of surgical instruments in his gynecological practice in the Quinta de Higiene. This event of 1890 occurred four short years after the first use of this method in Germany, and in 1892, the altruistic Santos Fernández gave the Hospital Mercedes (opened in 1882 replacing San Juan de Dios) its first modern oven for the preparation of surgical instruments.[10]

These were of course the Cuban dimensions of an applied scientific revolution that was everywhere shaking medicine.[11] Close on the heels of anesthesia, antiseptic and aseptic methodolgy made possible surgical procedures which were formerly impossible, or if possible, only practiced by the most daring or foolhardy. The conditions on the eve of this revolution are vividly described in a personal anecdote by J.A. Martínez-Fortún y Foyo:

> In 1866 . . . antisepsis was rudimentary, stoves were not used and almost all of the patients died of gangrene, tetanus, and other infections. In this year, my Aunt Angustias was given an operation by the famous Federico Gálvez, for a malignant maxilar tumor in a house on Havana Street with the back facing the alleyway "Espada." The operation was performed without taking off the black great coat that he used; he hardly washed his hands, with long yellow fingernails, with a simple washing of instruments; result, dead of tetanus in a few days. The sanitary conditions of the city were so bad that "there existed a cubic meter of fecal matter from black wells [crude cesspools]

in each sixty-two cubic meters of surface (La Guardia)." In these conditions, the Hospital "Reina Mercedes" was inaugurated . . . a hope in the midst of so many poor. To that date, only twenty abdominal operations had been practiced in Cuba with a mortality of almost 40%.[12]

Reflecting the advances in practical technology, dentistry emerged as a separate profession in the last half of the nineteenth century, with its own schools apart from the university by permission of the captain-general in 1879, the first year of peace after the Ten Years War, Cuba's long first war for independence. The first really proper dentists, from 1850 to 1860, were predominantly foreign—German and English but mostly North American—reflecting the proximity and early development of dentistry in the United States. Cubans who studied in New York, Philadelphia, Paris, or Switzerland joined with foreigners to open a number of dental schools, launch professional journals, and found the Dental Society, all shortly after 1879. The influx of foreign influences supplemented the continued use in Cuba of such texts as the *Manual of Bleeders and Dentists* (second edition), by Ambrosio González del Valle. The strong bonds between Cubans and Paris are seen in the *Anales de la Sociedad Ondontológica;* half of the articles solicited by the editors, Federico Poey[13] and Justiniani Chacón[14] were in French.[15]

Every large city of the interior had, by this time, developed a few families of medical patriarchs, such as the well-known Rubios, and Cuervos in Pinar del Río and the Martínez-Fortúns in Remedios. Improved transportation began to favor the work of physicians in the interior cities, especially in Matanzas, and the mushrooming size of sugar mills increased the demand for practitioners in those sites. Two theories might be suggested for the quality of the few physicians of the interior: Either they were slow to learn of new developments inaugurated in Havana, or, alternately, physicians of the interior included enough immigrants (like Carlos Finlay's father in Camagüey) and students returning from abroad so that medicine might have been equivalent or even better than that practiced in Havana. Whatever the truth of the matter, many legitimate practitioners are thought to have abandoned the interior in the wake of the last years of warfare, from 1895 to 1898. It is probable that medicine of the interior continued for some time as the medicine of the early nineteenth century. Late in the century, for example, the forces of the Liberation Armies included their barbers and bleeders, and, no doubt, a supply of folk healers.[16]

ECONOMY AND LIVING CONDITIONS

Sugar moved forward from 1823 to its golden age in the 1860s, accompanied by the illegal import of perhaps four hundred thousand slaves and the constant presence of some twenty-five thousand soldiers, as well as many civil guards or rural police. Trains appeared in 1837, and about 1840, functionally integrated sugar machines with vacuum boiling and centrifugal crystalization also appeared. Coffee lands turned over to sugar, but tobacco production increased throughout the century, with more tobacco workers in Havana in 1860 than today.[17]

War and Proletarianization

Unlike previous years, the period from 1868 to 1898 was studded with war and economic instability. Creole decadence partially gave way to an idealistic nationalism which was welded under arms, and under the collapse of public order, to a deeply popular, anti-Spanish movement of the predominantly black and mulatto poor. The sugar depression of the 1880s, followed by the destruction of the last war of independence, ruined many of the oligarchy, old aristocracy, and new bourgeoisie. Recovery inaugurated the industrial division of labor between capital-intensive sugar-processing plants called *centrales* and sugar farmers known as *colonos*, a name derived from the entrance of immigrant farmers into this specialty. The ultimate consequence of earlier and continuing efforts at white population development and of the final collapse of slavery (also in the 1880s), sugar production was rapidly proletarianized under the aegis of sugar corporations and *colonos*. The giant industrial mills, half of them owned by U.S. firms, were fed by rail networks, that finally destroyed the primitive mills that until recently had operated alongside the new. The observations offered in a previous section on the relationship between increased scale and instability on the one hand and work and living conditions on the other continue to apply then for the whole of the nineteenth century, notwithstanding the formal ending of slavery.

Social Class and the Medical Profession

In contrast to social class instability, the stability and lethargy of academic institutions, artificially protected from external forces, maintained a nostalgic air of aristocratic pretensions and a solemnity that dated from monastic origins. As the sons and daughters of the "better" classes turned in increasing numbers to medical and other professional, academic, and literary careers, they took from these areas intellectual and cultural prestige and added to them the aristocratic pretensions and sometimes the wealth of upper class origins. Upper class origins among physicians led to two tendencies in the profession. The freedom of some from material interests tended to preserve the intellectual and moral goals of medicine and also tended to encourage diversion from practical clinical work. As the effects of war, economic depression, and technological revolution threatened or ruined much of the sugar dependent classes in Cuba, displaced increasingly by foreign capital after 1880, many families maintained their social influence through the professions, the academy, and literary work. Alongside already established medical families, the tottering sugar oligarchy and declining aristocracy gave birth to medical dynasties which came to predominate among future names of Cuban medicine. In still another way the form of practice was influenced by the economic decline of old families. Private physicians who set up their offices in the old mansions of the rich acquired trappings of social class, as did the various *quintas* and *casas de salud*, mutualist and private, which were visible in the mid-nineteenth century and greatly developed in the 1880s.

HOSPITALS, CLINICS, AND MUTUALISM

The failure of public services to match the prosperity of sugar is suggested by the transfer in 1861 of four hundred patients from the collapsing general hospital, San Juan de Dios, to the upper floor of the Havana jail, thereafter a place to be avoided for its disgusting odor and appearance. The proximity of jail and hospital appropriately symbolize the conceptual proximity of the two custodial functions in the minds of Spanish administrators. When medical students were wounded by the Spanish mob in 1871, they were carried to the hospital rooms above the jail. The patrician friend of José Martí, Fermín Valdés Domínguez, later recalled the conditions: "I remember with horror the miserable ward of the hospital . . . without light, without air, without necessary cleanliness; the cots of cloth were heaped together and it was something other than a hospital . . . the sick were given a repugnant soup."[18]

Not until 1886 was the new city hospital building completed, this time renamed Nuestra Señora de Las Mercedes. The new building was constructed outside the suburbs of Havana, in the healthy site recommended years before by Romay for the quarantine lazareto of yellow fever patients. But the new "palace for the poor" was not connected to the city by an adequate road until an avenue expressly for that purpose was built by the government of the new republic. The only other significant hospital construction by the Spanish in Cuba were the military hospitals for the thousands of Spanish troops falling victim to yellow fever and other diseases. The Hospital Alfonso XII, near the present University of Havana, consisted of wooden barracks: fifty clinical rooms, twelve pavillions for infectious disease, four wards for officers, and six pavillions for convalescents. With the varied attentions of some twenty-seven practitioners and 170 other workers, the hospital treated 44,828 soldiers in 1897.[19] Renamed after a hero of independence, General Calixto García, the hospital was continued after the republic, variously rebuilt, and has served to the present as the principal university hospital. Other military hospitals were organized in the bare conditions of converted sugar warehouses, the principal one being in Regla.

During the urban concentration of the rural population under General Weyler, a makeshift emergency Hospital de Reconcentración was set up by civilians in Marianao. With the end of hostilities, in the same municipality, the Quinta Ofelia and the Las Merceditas ranch were turned into a veterans' hospital with the name Hospital Cubano. Of the same type were the Hospital Dóbroca on the Bocalandro ranch in San José de las Lajas, and the mansion hospital of the Filomeno coffee farm in Nuevo Paz.[20] But the only hospital established during the first intervention that afterward continued to exist was the Hospital Las Animas for infectious disease. A converted barracks for Spanish military engineers, it was soon dedicated exclusively to yellow fever patients and was the site of the famous studies of yellow fever by the United States Army Medical Commission.

Yellow Fever, Mutual Aid, and Hospitals

In some European cities, the appearance of syphilis is thought to explain the development of the urban hospital. Because the disease was neither limited to the lower classes nor "proper" for treatment in the home, it called for an institution with a curative bent. Yellow fever played a similar role in Cuban hospital history. Throughout the last half of the nineteenth century, this and other diseases and the inadequacy of public hospitals stimulated the formation of the small private infirmaries, *quintas*, or *casas de salud*. When mutual aid societies (stimulated partially by the compulsory return to Spain of indigent immigrants) were created among Spanish ethnic groups and certain occupational categories, the mutual aid societies were encouraged to develop group prepayment contracts with physicians and clinics and eventually to establish their own *quintas de salud*, even to hire their own physicians. (To some degree, disease no doubt played a role in the creation of the mutual aid societies in the first place.) By the end of the nineteenth century, the *quintas* of the principal Havana ethnic centers grew to hospital proportions, caring for their own members and new immigrants as well.

While, as we have seen, there were various mutualist endeavors in previous times, dating from the arrival of the very first trained physician, the first recorded mutualist *quinta* or clinic was a private venture launched in 1840 by a Frenchman, Francisco María Normand. Seeing the success of Belot's Casa de Salud in Regla, Normand established a vigorously competitive *quinta*, also in Regla, on property belonging to the physician Lorenzo Hernández, the son and heir of Belot's collaborator, the elder Lorenzo Hernández. Ambitiously advertising his services to the "business-

men of Havana, captains of ships, and to the general public," Normand offered lower prices and a prepaid subscription plan: seven pesos per man
per stay in Havana port for seamen (with private rooms for officers) and
one peso per month (one and a half for private rooms) for residents of
Havana and Regla. Home visits were also covered. Services to women
were offered on a fee-for-service basis in the home, but no women were
permitted in the Casa de Salud or covered by prepayment. (The same applied to all of the mutualist plans in the nineteenth century.) A free boat
was provided for transport between the clinic and the rail terminal to
Guanabacoa; surgical operations that were not covered by prepayment
would not be charged unless the patient completely recovered.

In the year following the opening of Normand's clinic, Belot closed his
Casa de Salud to join his son in a new ophthamology clinic in Havana; but
both facilities, Belot's and Normand's, were taken over by the Spanish
government to serve as places of compulsory quarantine. In 1875, the
leprosy hospital was moved to the old facility of the Normand clinic.[21]

By 1880, there were several private mutualist clinics in Havana, the
Clínica Mutualista of Gabriel Casuso y Roque, the Quinta de Garcini, and
the Quinta la Integridad Nacional. But the greatest growth in the last third
of the nineteenth century occurred in the clinics of the ethnic associations—
La Benéfica, La Covadonga, La Quinta del Rey, La Purísima Concepción, La
Castellana, La Balear, La Canaria, and others. It was these institutions that
were in a position, after the eradication of the diseases that propelled their
development, to turn their services to hospital and clinic-based medical
care, precisely at a time when the elements of modern medicine were
demanding an institutional setting. It happened thus that yellow fever, the
scourge of immigrants, shaped the peculiarly Cuban tendency toward the
domination of health care by mutualist, prepaid medicine, directed often by
lay organizations, and toward the general bias in favor of institutional settings for medical work. Many physicians early worked as employees in
hospitals and clinics, and even private physicians tended to seek clinics as
the favored setting for their practice. At the same time, it should be noted,
the specialization of yellow fever as a problem of immigrants prompted the
location of hospital services in or near the metropolitan ports.

Ironically, Cuban independence, economic recovery, and the eradication of yellow fever helped to stimulate even greater waves of emigration
from troubled Spain. The centros regionales, already prepared with
buildings, incentives, and organization, responded with greatly expanded
services. As hospital care became more integrated with general medical
care, the hospital and clinic services of the ethnic centers soon became their
most important function. Their growth constituted the largest institutional
development in medical services during the early national period. That this

development primarily benefitted the Spanish serves as an appropriately grotesque commentary on the new republic.

YELLOW FEVER AND WAR

Yellow fever, which remained the undaunted plague of foreign visitors,[22] was the greatest enemy of Spanish soldiers. The statistics on Spanish losses are startling. From 1895 to 1898, the Spanish employed over 200,000 troops in Cuba. For the distribution of casualities by rank and cause, see Table 4.1.

Table 4.1
Casualties of Spanish Troops
in Cuba by Rank and Cause, 1895-98*

	Killed in Battle	Died of Wounds	Died of Yellow Fever	Died of Other Diseases
Generals	1	—	—	—
Officers	81	463	313	127
Soldiers	704	8,164	13,000	40,000

*From Hugh Thomas, *Cuba: The Pursuit of Freedom*, New York: Harper and Row, 1971, p. 414.

Spanish deaths in the first war of independence or Ten Years War, from 1868 to 1878, were estimated by Spanish officials at 208,000, and might have revealed a similar distribution by rank and cause.[23] Knowing that officers enjoyed better living conditions and separate hospital facilities, the figures almost certainly reveal the extremely poor nutrition, sanitation, and hospital conditions of the troops.[24] The figures reveal the social class bias of the diseases involved, with less class discrimination by yellow fever than by other diseases. The category of "other diseases" included smallpox, malaria, tuberculosis, and dysentery. The ratio of "died of wounds" to "killed in battle" suggests the primitive state of military medicine and surgery. Spanish military physicians themselves fared only slightly better than other soldiers. Of 600 military physicians, who replaced civilian physicians in many towns of the interior, eight died of wounds compared to eighty who died of different diseases, including fifty who died of yellow fever.[25] Like officers, they were more susceptible to yellow fever and less susceptible to other diseases than were regular soldiers.

Yellow fever also offered the strongest military argument against United States intervention. Other diseases could supposedly be avoided by careful sanitary measures. Losses among U.S. troops in the Cuban intervention were the overwhelming consequence of yellow fever. Their distribution by rank and cause is shown in Table 4.2.

Table 4.2
U.S. Casualties by Rank and Cause, March-June 1898*

| | Officers | | | Men | | |
	Killed in Action	Died of Wounds	Died of Disease	Killed in Action	Died of Wounds	Died of Disease
Regulars	24	7	51	270	114	1,524
Volunteers	14	3	114	188	28	3,820
Totals	38	10	165	458	192	5,344

*From the *Report of the Adjutant General, 1898-99,* cited in Hugh Thomas, *Cuba: The Pursuit of Freedom,* New York: Harper and Row, 1971, p. 405.

Although the conditions are not precisely comparable, the much lower U.S. ratio of "died of wounds" to "killed in action" indicates the unquestionable superiority of U.S. military medicine and other health conditions, with the useful assistance of several Cuban physicians. The lower disparity among U.S. troops between disease mortality for officers and men than among the Spanish troops suggests a lower disparity between officers and lower ranks with respect to nutrition, sanitary conditions, and hospital care.

Civilian Mortality

The overwhelming weight of the war years fell heaviest, however, on the civilian population, where economic disruption aggravated already poor sanitary conditions. The most serious cause of civilian mortality was the rural concentration policy which was most notoriously effected in the second war period under the Spanish General Weyler. Given the epidemic conditions of Cuba and the clear sanitation and supply inabilites of the Spanish, the concentration orders, like the strategic hamlets and forced urbanization in Vietnam, amounted to a policy of extermination. Civilian losses were so great, especially affecting young children and the birth rate itself, that future census reports were always to be characterized by a reduced population in the relevant age groups. The losses have been estimated at 10 percent of the civilian population or around three hundred thousand in the years from 1895 to 1898.[26] A trench again had to be dug in the Havana cemetery for smallpox victims, while many died of starvation in the concentration camps.

In a sense, the war of independence was the long awaited slave uprising in Cuba. Perhaps 80 percent of the rebels were black or mulatto, including some of the most exceptional military leaders. The poorest sector in Cuba, the nonwhite population, also suffered most heavily. Their percentage of the population declined slightly and there were 20,000 fewer black and mulatto Cubans in the census of 1899 than in 1887, with more women than men![27] In addition to the effects of war, the living conditions of the black population declined after the official end of slavery in 1881.

FINLAY AND THE MOSQUITO THEORY

If yellow fever was important in hospital-clinic development and the enemy of soldier and immigrant, it was also the central concern of Cuban medicine and public health from the time of Romay.[28] The principal figure in this history, although often unrecognized as such, is the Cuban, Carlos J. Finlay. For his discovery[29] of the transmission of yellow fever by the *aedes aegypti* mosquito, Finlay's birthday came to be celebrated in Cuba as *el día del médico Cubano* and as *el día del médico americano* in Latin America. But the professional and official response to Finlay's discovery is hardly a matter for national pride. Finlay's work is a matter of embarrassment, not only for Cubans, but for Anglo-Americans as well. Although it seems inconceivable today, Finlay's discovery, announced in 1881, was for two decades rudely ignored and sometimes ridiculed by leading members of the medical profession in Cuba and the United States. While thousands died of yellow fever, Cubans, Spaniards and Anglo-Americans rejected—without research—Finlay's findings. Yet in 1901, one year after the practical implementation of Finlay's theory, Cuba was completely free of the dreaded disease.

Resistance to Finlay's Work

It is difficult to explain the seemingly irrational resistance to Finlay's work. A very important factor was the great enthusiasm of the time for germ theory and immunology. One might suppose, for instance, that the undevelopment of germ theory had made improbable, though not impossible, an early discovery of mosquito transmission by contemporaries of Romay. But the *development* of germ theory, while it hastened Finlay's discovery, simultaneously blinded his illustrious colleagues to the idea. Another factor would certainly be the commonplace and "harmless" nature of the insects themselves, although African slaves and Italian peasants had long regarded the mosquito as a source of illness. Above all, the failure was due to inadequate scientific methodology by Finlay's contemporaries and, partially, by himself. Moreover, Finlay's modest social background prejudiced some of his aristocratic or otherwise pretentious contemporaries against him.[30] Had a man such as Romay advanced the mosquito theory, its acceptance and implementation would certainly have been hastened by connections of social class, institutional position, and powerful friends. As it turned out, the promotion of the mosquito theory was begun by an unpretentious man of rather modest stature, socially *and* physically, for to make matters worse, Finlay periodically suffered from a stammering speech defect that derived from an attack of chorea in his childhood. At least one of Finlay's colleagues seriously protested that Finlay contradicted Romay's 1797 dissertation on yellow fever—a position that Romay himself later rejected! (So much for the destruction of sacred texts accomplished by Romay.) National chauvinism too played a deviously complex role. Some members of the academy were disdainful of Finlay's confidence in North American scientists, while among U.S. researchers it is undoubtedly the case that the universal chauvinism of Anglo-Americans toward the Cubans also affected their appreciation of Finlay's position. How ironic, therefore, that Finlay seemed foreign to Cubans (and to the Spanish) because he was the son of a Scottish eye surgeon! More directly political conflict may have been involved, although Finlay's political views seem to have gone unrecorded. An uncle gave aid to South American independence and a son, Frank, joined the Cuban independence army. Unlike his wife, the daughter of an Irish merchant, Finlay was only nominally Catholic.[31]

It is not as if few efforts were made by others to unlock the secrets of yellow fever. Five U.S. military medical commissions in Cuba, from 1879 to 1900, were dedicated to the objective of understanding its etiology and possible treatment. All of them failed, except for the last, which had as its sole objective the testing of Finlay's mosquito theory. The work of the U.S. Commission demonstrates the way in which attention was drawn from Finlay's theory by the fascination with narrow bacteriological and immunological approaches. Their aim was always the discovery of the "germ" of the disease, an interest which was further aggravated by the claims by the Italian, Saranelli, to have discovered the yellow fever bacillus. The energies of the U.S. Commission were directed toward disproving the Saranelli theory and other bacteriological theories while Finlay himself, without discounting his mosquito theory, also diffused his work in the search for the primary microbiological agent. When the U.S. Commission turned its attention, finally, to Finlay's mosquito theory, they were encouraged by the work of the British military surgeon, Ronald Ross, who had proven beyond doubt that malaria was transmitted by mosquitos.[32]

In 1898, Finlay joined the United States Army to aid in the liberation of Cuba, offering advice and clinical service, especially for yellow fever.

What Dr. William C. Gorgas said of U.S. sanitary efforts in 1901 could have been said of the Spanish after 1881. In a letter to Finlay, he said:

> What you say is very strong and perfectly true. If, when we went to Cuba, we had adopted your suggestions, the same results would have been accomplished in 1899 that were afterwards accomplished in 1901, and I would go further and say, as I believe, that it was through your work and personal advocacy of the mosquito theory that the American Board, of which Reed was Chairman, was induced to investigate the mosquito theory, and that if you had not have done the work which you had already done along these lines in 1900 the American Board would never have undertaken the investigation of the mosquito theory.[33]

The Mosquito Theory

The first U.S. Commission of 1879 was an important stimulus for Finlay's work. Until that time, he had sought climatological explanations for the disease and was conducting careful tests of the alkalinity of the atmosphere as a possible factor in the disease. His first published work on yellow fever in 1861 was almost identical to the point of view of Romay in 1820. He blamed stagnant waters, putrification, bad living, and so forth. Having evolved to a more precise climatological theory (against contagion), Finlay was influenced, probably by his associaton with the American bacteriologist Dr. George H. Sternberg, to see the validity of the arguments of the contagion position and the belief that the casual agent must be a microorganism. This led Finlay to the conclusion that there must be an intermediary vector which explained both positions. Observing a complete syndrome of contagion in a disease *foco*, why did a traveler so often fail to propagate the disease when, after departure from Havana, he fell ill with yellow fever in another port? Normal views of contagion were thus inadequate. But similar climates seemed to exist which did not give origin to the disease nor offer an environment for contagion. It was known that the disease could be innoculated from serum extracted from a victim of yellow fever. Why not consider the possibility that innoculation could be affected by the bite of a blood-sucking insect—perhaps the mosquito? Already suspecting the mosquito, Finlay announced his dialectical approach at the International Sanitary Conference in Washington, D.C., on February 18, 1881:

> We have on one side the contagionists and, on the other, the non-contagionists, each endeavoring to deny the importance of the cases brought forward by the contrary party in support of their respective opinions. Well, gentlemen, I declare that it is impossible for an impartial mind to look into the stated facts without arriving at the conclu-

sion that many of the proofs cited in favor of each of those two apparently contradictory opinions, must be accepted as perfectly authenticated facts, which conclusion necessarily leads to this other consequence, that we must admit the intervention of a third independent condition in order to account for those two orders of facts.

It is my personal opinion that three conditions are necessary in order that the propagation of yellow fever shall take place:

1. The presence of a previous case of yellow fever within certain limits of time . . . .

2. The presence of a person apt to contract the disease.

3. The presence of an agent entirely independent for its existence both of the disease and of the sick man, but which is necessary in order that the disease shall be conveyed from the yellow fever patient to a healthy individual.

It will be objected that this is a mere hypothesis; and indeed, it is only as such that I give it. But I believe it is a plausible one, which has, at least, the merit of explaining a certain number of facts which have remained hitherto unaccounted for by current theories. I do not ask for anything else, as my only object is to show that, if my hypothesis, or some other analogous to it, should be realized, all the measures which are now employed in order to disinfect and to check the progress of the disease would turn out to be without effect, in as much as the principal efforts should have been directed against the third condition, by endeavoring to destroy the agent of transmission or to divert it from the path that it follows in communicating the disease.[34]

Finlay's comment, we are told by a medical biographer, César Rodríquez Expósito, was given little attention by the conference and Finlay returned to Havana where he continued his work with his only collaborator, the Spanish physician Claudio Delgado. After careful studies of the *aedes aegypti*, Finlay attempted his first experimental test. A group of twenty nonimmunes, new Spainsh soldiers, were subjected to seven weeks of observation. Of these, five were made to be bitten on different occasions by different mosquitos that had previously bitten a yellow fever patient of the Quinta de Garcini. Of these men, three cases of yellow fever were diagnosed and one doubtful case was presented; of the remaining fifteen, no case of yellow fever was presented.[35]

On August 14, 1881, in a paper entitled "The Mosquito Hypothetically Considered as the Agent of Transmission of Yellow Fever," Finlay presented his finding to the Havana Academy of Sciences. Much of the supportive data for his theory was not new. A century earlier, commented Finlay, the most complete general treatment of the mosquito had been written by the French naturalist Reaumur, and in 1817 Felipe Poey carried some Cuban mosquitos to Paris where they were classified by Robineau Desvoidy, isolating the genus *culex mosquito (aedes agypti)*. "The need of an external intervention," added Finlay, "apart from the disease itself, in order that the latter may be transmitted is made apparent by numerous considerations; some of them already pointed out by Humboldt and Benjamin Rush since the beginning of the century." Conscious of the historical foundation and the role of his discovery, Finlay observed, "The application of the auxiliary sciences to Medicine often demands such a minute acquaintance with the different branches of human knowledge, that one cannot but wonder at the length of time which sometimes elapses before certain facts recorded in a special branch can become available for purely medical investigations." Integrating the wealth of accumulated knowledge, Finlay found his theory "strengthened by the numerous historical, geographical, entomological and meteorological coincidences which occur between the data . . . regarding the mosquito and those which are recorded about yellow fever; while at the same time, we are enabled by it [his theory] to account for circumstances which have until now been considered inexplicable under the prevailing theories."[36]

The findings presented, Finlay modestly concluded his model of scientific analysis:

These experiments are certainly favorable to my theory, but I do not wish to exaggerate their value in considering them final, although the accumulation of probabilities in my favor is now very remarkable. I understand but too well that nothing less than an absolutely incontrovertible demonstration will be required before most of my colleagues accept a theory so entirely at variance with the ideas which have until now prevailed about yellow fever . . . .

My only desire is that my observations be recorded, and that the correctness of my ideas be tested through direct experiments. I do not mean by this that I would shun the discussion of my opinion; far from it, I shall be very glad to hear any remarks or objections which my distinguished colleagues may be inclined to express.[37]

The remarkable presentation was received with cold indifference by the members of the academy. Not a single question was asked, not a single clarification requested![38] For years Cuba awaited this discovery, but the mosquito theory waited twenty years for acceptance.

FINLAY'S EARLY WORK

Finlay's work is of great interest when it is considered as a stimulus which might reveal the character of its environment. In this regard, Finlay's early career is in some respects more revealing and perhaps more brilliant than his work on yellow fever. Without the context of his previous work, Finlay's work on yellow fever is easily made to seem like an accidental observation by an otherwise irrelevant physician. Nothing could be farther from the truth. Finlay's discovery of yellow fever transmission was the logical development of a career dedicated to the methods of science in medicine. An opthamologist and eye surgeon in his father's footsteps, Finlay, like other great discoverers, made contributions to areas that were marginal to his specialty.

Cholera

Well acquainted with research on cholera, Finlay first published in 1865 or 1866 a paper in the annals of the Academy of Science which offered a summary discussion of the etiology and treatment of the disease. His father had also specialized in its treatment in Camagüey after its appearance in Cuba in 1833. When, in 1867, cholera was again epidemic in Havana, Finlay tried to understand the course of the disease by employing the epidemiological model used in London in 1865 by John Snow. Snow, known to some as the founder of modern epidemiology, had demonstrated independently of germ theory, that the London epidemic stemmed from water sources. Finlay charted the address, distance from the Zanja Real (water supply canal), and time of attack for 130 victims of cholera, of whom at least 91 died, in the Cerro suburb of Havana from November 11, 1867, to January 29, 1868. Through the Cerro ran the water supply canal, an open ditch from the Almendares River. After cholera first broke out in another part of the city, with 120 cases in the city's hospitals, Finlay determined to replicate the finding reported in other countries, that cholera "runs downhill." In a letter offered for publication in the *Diario de la Marina* in June 1868, Finlay presented his analysis and offered popular advice for control of cholera:

> The first cases observed in the Cerro were two blacks taken ill while they were cleaning the filters of the Zanja; . . . there occured two more that day and the next in the home where the two mentioned blacks had rested, and from the thirteenth . . . other cases occurred, the epidemic propagating itself not from one house to the next, but in houses distant from one another, but situated over the Zanja or that received some of its uncovered branches.
>
> But at this moment the epidemic reigns in Mazorra, very close to the Rio Almendares, for which motive I believe it is to the point to recommend to the authorities that they not permit that . . . the neighbors of this locality spill the cholerous virus into the water of the river, washing clothes or other contaminated objects, because the morbid

cause would surely be taken toward Puentes Grandes and through "los Filtros" (insufficient for the matter) to the Zanja and with this to the Cerro and other sections of Havana.[39]

The letter was not published; the official censor apparently interpreted the letter as a critique of the Spanish administration which had not been able to combat the epidemics of cholera. Finally, in September 1873, Finlay found opportunity to present in the Academy of Science a technical review of the work on cholera by Snow in England, Pettenkoffer in Germay, Robin in France, and others—along with his own research. Finlay's presentation, and the somewhat hostile discussion recorded in the *Annals* of the academy, give a picture of the sanitary conditions of the time. The ensuing debate on the potability of the water of the Zanja is one of the most interesting exchanges within the academy, occupying at least seven sessions between September 28, 1873, and February 8, 1874.

The Zanja Real was constructed over some fifty years at the end of the seventeenth century. Finlay cited Pezuela:

The work was reduced to a wide trench which brought almost undrinkable water during the rainy season, and which had to be repaired constantly . . . In 1833-34 it was again reconstructed to improve the condition of the water destined for public consumption, although that which is brought by la Zanja serves almost exclusively for irrigation and washing; because after the construction of the Aqueduct it continued coming as before, uncovered and almost always dirty . . . and carrying strange bodies and filth.[40]

The discussion in the academy revealed that in the first epidemic of 1833 and 1834, the majority of cases occurred outside the walls of the city, which were served, for the greater part, by the Zanja. At least two doctors, Abreu and Gutiérrez, had at that time qualified its waters as unhealthy. In the interior of the city, people enjoyed somewhat safer water supplies, served frequently by wells, cisterns, or the aqueduct. But the expanding population of the Cerro greatly aggravated hazardous conditions. Many extensions of the main water channel were cut, permitting the waters to flow under many houses, near others, and even under a new match factory. Vessels of all kinds, from the bedroom, kitchen, and latrine were washed in its open waters.

"Also," added Finlay, "I will mention the general use that is made of the water of the Zanja by the milkmen to wash their bottles and sometimes perhaps to adulterate the milk."[41]

The counterarguments, led by the president of the academy, Ambrosio González del Valle and the somewhat more sophisticated vice-president, Dr. Babé, rested upon the "test of time" that had proclaimed the water drinkable. Warning against "mere statistics" and against the "autocracy of chemistry," the microscope was declared unready to resolve every problem of epidemic. Chemistry without physiology (Ambrosio González del Valle's field) was meaningless, they said. Besides, said Ambrosio, the waters of the Zanja continue to supply "the students of the Colegio de Carraguao, the neighbors of the Cuartel de Madera . . . the Quinta de Garcini, and . . . the ice factory that services all the cafés and restaurant stands of the city, without any risk at all to health[!]" To this questionable observation, Finlay wisely retorted that the issue was not whether the Zanja was poisonous but simply whether the water was healthy. On the seventh day of discussion the official conclusion of the Academy was, however, to declare the water of the Zanja safe for drinking.[42]

One explanation of the twisted conclusion of the academy is suggested by a casual comment by Finlay's opposition: to declare the water unhealthy might reinforce a popular belief that material found in the water was derived from dead Chinese and Africans. But the underlying issue was the reputation of the Spanish government (busy fighting the Cuban revolutionary armies from 1868 to 1878). A stamp of "unhealthy" or "undrinkable" on the water of the Zanja Real might have exacerbated social instability or even caused a wave of hysteria, always feared in epidemics. An increased demand on the preferred sources of water could have overburdened the more hygienic sources of the city and caused shortages for the entire population. Meanwhile, the officials felt no great urgency, since the better classes of Havana drank from the preferred sources. Why, Finlay somewhat peevishly asked, if the waters of the Zanja were so good, did everyone so clearly prefer for themselves the water of the aqueduct?

Other Medical Debates

Cholera provided but the most important of many examples of conflict between Finaly's statistical and scientific method and the sophistry and unrestrained personal interests of his contemporaries. A few other issues may be briefly mentioned. Against Finlay's condemnation of the unsafe and unhygienic conditions of a Havana soap factory, a Dr. Rovira argued for the narrow interests of industry, protesting that it had not been proven that industrial smoke could be hazardous to the health of a community.[43] Contrasted with Finlay's scientific argument in favor of compulsory sequestration of lepers based on the possibility of contagion, del Valle regarded sequestration justified merely by the repulsive nature and lack of social utility of lepers, "the rich sequestering themselves and the society sequestering the poor." (Interestingly, Finlay anticipated his approach to yellow fever contagion by suggesting in the case of leperosy that an intermediary factor, related to climate or geography might influence the efficiency of contagion.)[44] Even Finlay's position in favor of strenuous physical exercise as a postitive health measure in warm climates was in variance with a popular view expressed in the medical press. In terms reminiscent of medieval medicine, the arguments against Finlay clumsily reinforced the prevailing aristocratic disdain for manual labor and physical exercise in a society that had so degraded labor by human slavery.[45] High risk surgical intervention was simplistically opposed by many, while Finlay looked to statistical evidence for direction in such matters. Even the prestigious Dr. Juan Santos Fernández, the editor of the *Boletín Clínico Quirúrgico* and founder of the Havana Society for Clinical Studies, committed a travesty on science when he published without revision an article authored by himself which had previously been shown by Dr. Finlay to include dangerous clinical errors.[46] Finally, as slavery approached its end in Cuba, frail efforts were made to resurrect the long discredited, but still powerful, theory of the inhospitality of Cuba for population by Europeans. In opposition, Finlay painstakingly analyzed mortality tables to show that when allowance was made for an initial susceptibility to yellow fever, Cuba was as healthy as various countries of Europe that enjoyed that reputation.[47]

Finlay's conflicts with the medical hierarchy were not restricted to debate. In 1853, Finlay was refused admission to the University of Havana Medical School and enrolled in Jefferson Medical College in Philadelphia.[48] Graduating in 1855 and returning to Cuba, the Spanish-Cuban authorities refused to validate his degree. The Academy of Sciences, for seven years after 1864, denied full membership to Finlay. The subject of his thesis presented in solicitation of membership was, again ironically, the etiology of yellow fever!

What, in sum, does Finlay's experience tell us about late nineteenth century Cuban medicine? Finlay himself offers the best answer in an 1876 speech to the Academy of Sciences on the occasion of its fifteenth anniversary. Two years after the dismal discussion of cholera transmission in Havana water supply, his speech was a partially disguised but constructive attack on the perversion of science within the academy. The speech is important for raising the conflict from the area of specific problems to a conflict within the technology of science itself:

Those who censure the use of hypotheses and preconceived ideas in the experimental method, have fallen in the error of confusing the invention of the experiment with the observation of its results. It is reasonably said that the results of the experiment should be observed with the mind stripped of hypotheses and preconceived ideas. But one must take much care to not proscribe the use of hypotheses or of ideas when it is a matter of instituting an experiment or of imagining means of observation. One ought to the contrary give free course to imagination; the idea is the beginning of all reasoning and of all invention, from which flows every kind of initiative. One must not suffocate nor reject it under the pretext that it might be harmful, for it only needs to be regulated and given criteria, which is very different.[49]

In short, the scientific revolution had rescued the Cuban medical academy from speculative scholasticism only to have it fall into crude empiricism, clinical individualism, and mindless data collection. The weapons of antischolasticism were being turned against speculation itself!

UNITED STATES INTERVENTION

Medical hierarchies were not fundamentally changed with the coming of independence. Just as the military governor ruled with slightly modified Spanish administrative structures, so the medical and dental societies reemerged under members already prominant, if not dominant, in the 1880s and 1890s. Under General Wood's government, Santos Fernández became president of the Academy of Sciences, now housed in a new building. Finlay, by way of his new fame, became Director of Sanitation. (While his old antagonist, Ambrosio González del Valle was relegated to a small municipal direction of sanitation.) The first Cuban Medical Congress held in 1890 had been presided by Joaquín Albarrán; in 1905 the first National Cuban Medical Congress was presided by Joaquín's brother Pedro.[50] Some new faces appeared in the services of sanitation and hospitals and acquired prestige from the extraordinary success in both areas. Key posts were filled by Cubans who had previously taken up careers in the United States and, quite secondly, by Cubans active in the Liberation Army. Almost all of the circle of physicians who integrated the pro-independence groups in the United States or who held positions in the early military sanitation efforts found themselves in key sanitary and hospital posts for the rest of their lives.[51] Although the principle losers were the Spanish, they were not systematically ostracized from the lower bureaucracies until the Liberal and nationalist government of José Miguel Gómez set a decidedly anti-Spanish course in 1909.

Eradication of Yellow Fever

The contributions of the U.S. medical commission and the new Department of Sanitation under the North American occupation were profound. Controlled experiments proved, although many physicians were yet unconvinced, that yellow fever was transmitted by the *aedes aegypti* mosquito. Armed with these findings, United States Army surgeons and a corps of Cuban physicians and health workers supplemented Finlay's sanitary recommendations with an efficient campaign organized along military lines, not altogether different from public health campaigns in socialist Cuba today. Three brigades of mosquito workers were organized. The Segomya Brigade, the name then given to the *aedes aegypti* mosquito, worked in the central sections of Havana. The Anopheles Brigade was organized to work in the suburbs where the *anopheles* mosquito, the vector in malaria contagion, was more commonly found. And the third, Yellow Fever Brigade, had the task of exterminating mosquitos infected by victims of yellow fever.

The results were dramatic. In early 1901 almost all of Havana's 26,000 houses had been found to be active breeding grounds for the *aedes aegypti*. The uncovered receptacles and open cesspools found in most homes offered themselves everywhere to the mosquito. By the end of the year, only 290 of 16,121 houses inspected in December were found to have mosquito larvae. In the suburbs, ditches were dug to drain pools and swamps. Yellow fever patients were immediately isolated in carefully screened rooms and great quantities of pyrethrum powder were used used to exterminate mosquitos in nearby dwellings. Such measures were assisted by a vigorous program of health propaganda. The preceding thirty years had produced an average yearly mortality rate by yellow fever in Havana of 706. In 1900 mortality reached 310, but in 1901 yellow fever claimed only 18 deaths, of which 13 occurred before the mosquito work began, with the last case registered in September. Deaths from malaria declined significantly from a previous average of 513 and a mortality of 344 in 1900 to 151 deaths in 1901.[52]

In related matters, many roads and bridges were built, public buildings rebuilt, and municipalities reorganized. Hospitals were renovated in Santiago, Sancti Spíritus, Camagüey and other interior cities, while Mercedes in Havana, quite new to begin with, was completely overhauled, receiving not only a magnificent new operating facility but also a new sewage line.[53] A school of nursing, Cuba's first, was established in the Mercedes Hospital with nurses from the United States serving as its first instructors. Its first students graduated in 1902. Through careful control of horses, the epidemic incidence of glanders[54] was virtually eliminated in Havana. A program of smallpox vaccination was undertaken, also with characteristic military discipline, reducing to near zero the number of cases in Havana in 1901. An antituberculosis campaign, largely educational in nature, was begun, and plans were made for tuberculosis sanitorium. A department of sanitation and a department of charities (including hospitals) was reestablished as in Spanish days under the secretary of the interior.

Governor General Leonard Wood reported on the successful work of 1901:

> The hospitals throughout the Island are in excellent condition. Well equipped and supplied with all necessary apparatus and supplies. Training school for nurses under the direction of the best nurses procurable in the United States have been established in connection with nearly all of the large hospitals. Cuba today is far better supplied with hospital facilities than most of our country outside of the immediate vicinity of the larger cities. Large sums have been spent in this work, but the beneficient results have been very great. The work done has enabled the methods of modern surgery and the modern treatment of diseases to be established in Cuba and in a year conditions have been advanced from those of 50 years ago to modern conditions.[55]

The achievements of public health efforts under United States occupation were not the simple consequence of "Yankee organization." An essential ingredient was the liberation of new Cuban energies, optimism and motivation. Fortún y Foyo recalls the era as "a period of enthusiasm and hope," and Dr. José A. López del Valle, remembering his work as the young director of disinfection in the first (U.S.-Cuban) Department of Sanitation, adds:

> If we are to faithfully fulfill our mission as impartial historians, we ought to confess that in these first instances, there was neither uniform plan nor did there exist methods of work, nor firm and sure scientific direction. The good intentions of everyone, of those who ordered and of those who were to obey, was that which filled these empty holes and lack of organization.[56]

The first intervention, then, was a kind of breathing period, in which the ambiguities of independence under U.S. paternalism and economic domination waited beneath the surface. The great ideological and civil leader, José Martí, was dead, with no other figure to command unity. Gone also were the much loved and ideologically astute generals, José and Antonio Maceo and Calixto García. Other army leaders, denied normal acknowledgment by U.S. officials, were incompletely disarmed, inadequately rewarded by position or wealth, and their army yet unpaid. Meanwhile economic recovery began, with profits going to U.S. investors and again to Spanish merchants. Everyone was encouraged to seek personal profit from improving conditions, while the U.S. administration, on the heels of the corrupt Spanish, failed to present a sufficiently inspiring example of selfless service. An astute note of apprehension crept into Wood's glowing report of 1901 (emphasis added):

The affairs of this department while under the direction of Major Kean have been very largely influenced by a central board composed of Cuban gentlemen of intelligence and energy, representing the various provinces of the Island. They have all taken great interest in the work and I believe will continue to maintain it to the best of their ability after the withdrawal of our government. Of course, *if the coming government does not systematically support this department, it is bound to go under because the municipalities will not be sufficiently developed and public sentiment sufficiently educated and organized* to maintain a system which has brought so many benefits to the sick and suffering of the Island.[57]

THE NEW REPUBLIC

The first Cuban government of Tomás Estrada Palma failed to inspire many Cubans. The legislature was inactive and the government had little military or police strength. From the more or less centralized government of intervention, there emerged a regionally and ideologically fragmented state, its responsible public services predominating in Havana alone. The administration of public health inherited from General Wood, already strongly decentralized into municipal finance and control, failed precisely as Wood had anticipated. Although a brilliant sanitation code was drafted under Finlay's direction, the responsibility for its promotion rested with local boards. There existed an extreme scarcity of competent personnel, support, and organization, with sufficient motivation and understanding to overcome such difficulties. Moreover, the work of sanitation and hospitals was divided as in recent Spanish times into separate departments of the secretary of the interior. Although not wrong in principle, the work was sometimes further confused by the overlapping authority that was exercised by the Junta Superior de Sanidad and Junta Superior de Beneficencia, boards which included representatives from many related institutions: the Special Commission on Hygiene (formerly the Yellow Fever Commission), the Academy of Sciences, the Sociedad Patriótica, the Medical School, the League Against Tuberculosis, and representatives from the east of Cuba, the west, and from Havana. Thus, administrative decisions could be made without operative responsibilities or accountability. César Rodríguez Expósito writes:

The Sanitary Organization that was established with the Republic was in theory perfect, but in practice it resulted in great and rocky difficulties, since the Local Boards remained inactive, for not having economic resources. The outfitting, staff, and hygienic attentions ceased to be offered. In Havana the same did not happen, for as the unique exception, the State continued attending the economic part of the expenses of sanitation.[58]

In health, as in other matters, the new Cuban government proved itself first of all the government of Havana.

Well-Intentioned Efforts

To well-intentioned officials part of the answer lay in the direction of greater centralization. Efforts of this kind, though unsuccessful in the Cuban legislature, were finally realized by decree of the second U.S. intervention, which restored order after the Liberal uprising against the dishonest elections organized by Estrada Palma. Sanitation and Charities were joined under a single cabinet level ministry, with mere advisory power given to a Junta Superior de Sanidad y Beneficencia. Local health posts were to be centrally appointed.

The greatest idealism lay behind this development. Pedro Albarrán exhorted the Cuban Congress:

The right to exist, the right to live, is necessarily anterior to all other rights of man. The state has the obligation of guaranteeing this right before all others. A considerable number of diseases that threaten man's existence can be prevented; therefore each citizen has the right to demand of their government that they be preserved from them, taking the necessary measures . . . The administration of Public Hygiene requires, by its special nature, uniformity of scientific criterion and perfect unity of action on the part of those responsible . . . without which . . . the necessary results will never be completed, no matter how good and wise the laws may be.[59]

The great difficulties and limitations of reorganization were also predictable. Against the proposed ministry, Méndez-Capote argued:

The Secretariat of Sanitation and Charity should not be founded to create and regulate that which is not yet constituted as habits and customs of our own; this is painful to say, but why must it not be confessed, modern hygiene is unknown even among many physicians.

The organization of the Secretariat . . . will not be other than the establishment of one more bureaucratic Center, a useless obstruction in the path of the State.[60]

As another legislator happily pointed out, raising the bureaucratic status did not increase the budget. The second medical revolution made possible the social idealism expressed by Albarrán, a far cry from the wholly paternalistic social morality of Romay, but implementation was frustrated by countless barriers. Méndez-Capote, who spoke against the new ministry, later became its secretary while his brother, a lawyer, became vice-president of the republic.

The odor of corruption was never far away. Governor Magoon failed in the second U.S. intervention of 1907 to require sufficient record-keeping of fines levied against sanitary violators. In his first circular to local chiefs, the aging Finlay ominously ordered them to not appoint friends or relatives as sanitary inspectors.[61] Corrupt patronage found few real limits. When Juan Guiteras took over from Finlay, he immediately presented his resignation to protest the extension of political appointments from the sphere of sanitation to the direction of hospitals. His resignation not accepted, Guiteras's determined action must have won concessions, but his influence probably did not greatly extend beyond his own professional fiefdom in the Las Animas Hospital. Here Guiteras served as director after 1903 until he accepted the position of Secretary of Sanitation and Charities in the cabinet of President Zayas in 1921. (In the meantime Guiteras also served as president of the Commission on Infectious Diseases after 1902; spokesman for Western Cuba on the Superior Board of Sanitation, 1903-1909; dean of the university medical faculty, 1905-1909; and director of sanitation, 1909-1913.) But men like Guiteras, always overextended, who sought to establish a purely technical administration in health affairs, were no match for the financial limitations and pressures against them. In 1925, in a letter to a Cuban journalist, Guiteras recalled:

> The position of Director of Sanitation had to clash at each step with the impossibility which our government leaders always encountered in order to be able to declare that the Secretariat of Sanitation is a technical organization which should only take into account the interests of Sanitation itself. And who impeded the leaders from making such declaration? Well, everyone, almost everyone.[62]

Guiteras is representative of the Cubans of good family who increasingly remained disdainfully above politics, that group who—often highly educated, altruistic, and clinging to aristrocratic notions and also to bureaucratic, academic, or professional posts—nonetheless were constantly compromised by their less principled compatriots. The government of Zayas proved to be even more corrupt than those of Gómez or Menocal. Guiteras, aging and unskilled in administrative details, was sacrificially dismissed to make way for the "honest cabinet" that was imposed upon Zayas by U.S. Consul Enoch Crowder.

Decline of Public Expectations

These observations signal the decline of great expectations for early national institutions. The first years of the republic inaugurated corrupt practices that were variously regarded as commonplace through the end of the presocialist period. Reinaugurated might be more accurate, of course, since many kinds of corruption were long common under Spanish rule. Bribes were often the key to hospital admission, guaranteed public services, and finding and keeping certain employment. Mosquito control programs gained notoriety as political pork barrel or outright fraud. In an island free of snakes, *matando la culebra*, killing snakes, became the euphemism for such work. As positions came to be regarded as sinecures or as old-fashioned personal property, they were frequently rented to substitutes (an old Spanish practice banned by Wood). When governments changed, bureaucracies were reshuffled, calling for new bribes, negotiations, and compromises. This fact, which weighed heavily on responsible physicians and others, caused instability and discontinuity which, anticipating more of the same, encouraged a kind of frenetic unaccountability that became characteristically Cuban, while hardly unique to that country.

It is not difficult to imagine the consequences that such processes held for the quality of services rendered, or for the balance between services and the monies allocated for them by government. The reputation of government-related employment and official duties declined, causing physicians who had a real choice to be dissuaded from such work.

Other Institutional Developments

While responsible government work in public health declined, the important medical efforts lay elsewhere. Private practice, as always, followed money, and now more than ever money was in Havana. Dámaso Lainé took advantage of a brilliant medical career in the United States and established in a fashionable suburb his Clínica Anglo-Americana, which catered to the small North American colony and wealthy Cubans. The bourgeoning Spanish immigrants were served by the Quinta Covadonga of the Centro Asturiano and by other *quintas de salud*.[63] A significant development in the medical school was the new specialty of tropical medicine which, in the spirit of independence, began slowly to focus attention on inglorious, but widespread, Cuban problems of intestinal parasitism and gastroenteritis. Under the influence of Finlay's triumph and the continued efforts against malaria and for the general sanitation, this specialty manifested the beginnings of an environmental and social approach to disease and health that was quite at odds with the glossy breakthroughs in clinical areas, dominant in every medical school of the time, not excepting the University of Havana.

While more physicians became employees of institutions, the tuition to medical and dental schools was cut in half by the first liberal government. But the mildly reformed structure of the university, somewhat crowded with students, did not provide improved preparation or possibilities for graduation. Thus, a small incident in the medical school prompted the formation of the Federation of University Students in 1921. This event, stimulated by a growing Latin American movement for university reform, expressed both dissatisfaction with authoritarian professors and disillusionment with government under the former exponents of independence. It pointed the way to the autonomy of the university and also to greater autonomy of the professions.

Thus, the great and revolutionary changes in health and health protection ushered in at the turn of the century quickly faded from view in the new dynamics of status quo in the new republic. These dynamics are revealed in the growing conflicts experienced by Cuban physicians: with the university as students, with the ethnic centers as employees and as competitors, with the government as employees and as an interest group, and with other physicians as competitors for employment, position, and patients. These conflicts, falling out of the independence period, grew sharply, expressing themselves in the forms that are here regarded as the third revolution in Cuban medicine. Finlay, in retrospect, was oddly marginal not only before but *after* he was finally acclaimed for his epochmarking work. This marginality is probably a sign, not only of the weakness of prerevolutionary medicine, but also of the weaknesses within the second revolution itself. Brilliant advances were made in clinical and social medicine at the turn of the century, yet they remained divided, the latter eclipsed rapidly by the former. The gleaming objects that were the site of the new clinical medicine became the constant preoccupation of physicians and laymen alike.

NOTES

1. In the González del Valle y Cañizo family there was, in addition to Fernando, at least two others in the nineteenth century university: Esteban G. del Valle y Cañizo, who held a professorship in philosophy (known also as "Aristotelian Text"), and Ambrosio G. del Valle y Cañizo, who later became president of the Academy of Sciences. (See Le Roy y Gálvez, p. 10.) In twentieth-century Cuba, the same family, it seems, was regarded as millionaires, having provided the funds for the founding of a religious private school. (Personal communication with José Moreno, University of Pittsburgh, 1973.)

2. The ring, book, and sword were given to the new doctorate by the dean of the faculty in an elaborate graduation ceremony that ended in a formal procession to the Cathedral where an oath was sworn before the bishop. The licenciate involved a similar ceremony, a custom which continued after the "secularization" of the university in 1842. See, for example, Le Roy y Gálvez, pp. 38-50.

3. His protector, Professor José Benjumeda, found himself forced to resign

from his professorship when a law of 1855 made the simultaneous holding of his post with the Military Sanitary Corps incompatible with university appointment. See Le Roy y Gálvez, p. 53.

4. In the public competition for the post of assistant, his only adversary was Ambrosio González del Valle y del Cañizo. Consequently, two positions were awarded rather than one. Ibid., p. 24.

5. Ibid., p. 44.

6. Ibid., p. 46.

7. *Voluntarios* were vigilantes from the Spanish immigrant community who were recruited to fight Cuban insurgents.

8. Bustamente was then professor of anatomy. Unsurprisingly, the anatomy courses were soon removed to the old Hospicio de San Isidro and no records of the event were allowed to remain in the university. Ibid., pp. 69-87.

9. José A. Martínez-Fortún y Foyo, p. 28.

10. Ibid., p. 27.

11. An excellent treatment of these developments is found in a chapter entitled "The Bacteriological Era and its Aftermath" in George Rosen, *A History of Public Health* (New York: MD Publications, 1958), pp. 294-336.

12. Martínez-Fortún y Foyo, p. 25.

13. Federico Poey was the son of Felipe Poey, the famous naturalist, university professor (for many years), and contemporary of Romay. Felipe was in turn the son of one of the late eighteenth century French-Cuban slaving enterprises, "Poey and Hernández," who later appeared in the ranks of large mill owners. See Thomas, p. 83.

14. While Poey studied in Paris and Geneva, the aristocratic Chacón was known as "the dentist from New York." (Martínez-Fortún y Foyo, pp. 21-22.)

15. Ibid., p. 30.

16. See César Rodríguez Expósito, "Indice de médicos, dentistas, farmacéuticos y estudiantes en la guerra de los diez años," *Cuadernos de Historia de Salud Pública, no. 40* (Havana: Ministerio de Salud Pública, 1968).

17. Thomas, p. 134.

18. del Pino y de la Vega, p. 33, citing a quotation in Luis A. de Arce, *Nuestra Señora de las Mercedes, 1597-1952, Historia de un hospital* (Havana: Editorial Selecta, 1952), p. 30.

19. del Pino y de la Vega, p. 43.

20. Ibid., pp. 47-48.

21. Gómez Luaces, pp. 40-45. Lepers rioted to protest harsh conditions under the early republic; they were moved to Rincón, where a leper asylum continues to function, mainly for the aged.

22. Havana registered 32,664 deaths from yellow fever in the years 1856-1905, with one year claiming over 2,000 and thirteen years with 1,000 or more deaths. Since yellow fever was endemic in Havana, taking a mild infantile form, many of the deaths were probably foreign. But when yellow fever passed to nonimmune nations, the numbers of dead were staggering. See Carlos E. Finlay (son of Carlos J. Finlay), *Carlos Finlay and Yellow Fever* (New York: Oxford University Press, 1940), p. 48 and pp. 164-65. See also Erwin H. Ackernecht, *History and Geography of the Most Important Diseases,* (New York: Hafner, 1965), pp. 50-59.

23. Thomas, p. 414.

24. Comparing the conditions of the makeshift character of most Spanish army hospitals, del Pino y de la Vega notes that officers were often given special entrance to the old San Ambrosio, where they enjoyed iron beds with mosquito nets. (del Pino y de la Vega, p. 43.)

25. Martínez-Fortún y Foyo, p. 30.

26. Thomas, p. 423.

27. Ibid., p. 429.

28. See Romay, vol. 1, pp. 65-107. Treatment changed little, it seems, until after 1860, for there was still much blood-letting in 1841. See de Acer, *El Real Hospital Nuestra Señora del Pilar*, p. 85, for a description of cures.

29. Finlay was the first to state the hypothesis concerning transmission of yellow fever by the mosquito, but he did of course have precursors, and undoubtedly to his greater credit, he must have made use of their work. He was less a discoverer than a researcher and advocate for a theory. See discussion in Ackerknecht, p. 58 and Moll, pp. 239-40.

30. His father, Edward, a Scottish eye surgeon with clinical training in the Hotel Dieu of Paris, established himself in Camagüey and later moved his practice to Havana. It is said that Edward Finlay had been bound originally, like his brother, to give assistance to the independence struggles in South America but, shipwrecked in Trinadad, he was married to a French woman. Neither did Carlos marry a nice Cuban girl; rather he married Adela Shine, the daughter of an Irish merchant in Cuba. In addition to a biography written by his son (cited above), see "Finlay" by César Rodríguez Expósito in Finlay, *Obras completas*, pp. 19-84.

31. This is my guess, in as much as he did not attend religious services, but his religious views, like his political views, do not seem to be recorded. See Carlos E. Finlay, p. 27.

32. See Ackerknecht, p. 98.

33. The document is reproduced in a collection of relevant material. See *Dr. Carlos J. Finlay and the "Hall of Fame" of New York*, Booklet on Sanitation History, no. 15, (Havana: Ministry of Health and Hospital's Assistance, 1959), p. 73.

34. Carlos J. Finlay, *Obras completas*, vol. 1, pp. 197-98.

35. Ibid., pp. 274-75.

36. Ibid., p. 273.

37. Ibid., pp. 275-76.

38. Rodríguez Expósito in Ibid., p. 41.

39. Carlos J. Finlay, vol. 3, pp. 396-97.

40. Ibid., p. 410.

41. Ibid., p. 403.

42. Ibid., pp. 429-43.

43. Ibid., pp. 553-54, pp. 563-68.

44. Ibid., p. 574.

45. Ibid., pp. 543-48.

46. See Ibid., pp. 511-24 and pp. 529-34.

47. Carlos J. Finlay, vol. 1, pp. 143-81.

48. A proper biography would here examine Finlay's relation to other developments in science and philosophy. It is interesting to note that at Jefferson Medical

College, Finlay studied closely with disciples of the Frenchman, Claude Bernard, an outstanding biologist and physiologist who is also remembered as a "materialist" theoretician of scientific method.

49. Carlos J. Finlay, vol. 3, p. 495.

50. J.A. Martínez-Fortún y Foyo, *Apuntes*, pp. 26, 34.

51. Well known names are: José A. López del Valle, Arístedes Agramonte, Juan Guiteras, Enrique Barnet, and Jorge Le Roy. See César Rodríguez Expósito, "La primera secretaria de sanidad del mundo se creó en Cuba," *Cuadernos de Historia de Salud Pública,* no. 25 (Havana: Ministerio de Salud Pública, 1964).

52. W. C. Gorgas, "Statement on Yellow Fever and the Mosquito," in *Dr. Carlos Finlay and the "Hall of Fame of New York,"* pp. 57-63.

53. An extensive source on physical conditions in Cuba, together with many photographs, budgetary, and engineering details, is the *Report of Major W. M. Black, Corps. of Engineers, U.S.A., Chief Engineer, Department of Cuba, for the Six Months ending December 31, 1900 (Civil Report of Major General Wood on Cuba, 1900).* The facilities of the Havana Jail (San Juan de Dios was on the top floor, 1868-1882) and the Mercedes hospital are described in great detail. See pp. 322-23 and pp. 387-97.

54. A contagious disease of horses occasionally transmitted to humans, with high fever, swelling of glands in the neck, and often death.

55. Leonard Wood, *Report of the Military Governor*, p. 45, pages reproduced in *Dr. Carlos Finlay and the Hall of Fame of New York*, pp. 49-54.

56. Cited in Rodríguez Expósito, "La primera secretaria de sanidad," p. 10.

57. Wood, p. 45, copied in *Dr. Carlos Finlay and the Hall of Fame of New York*, p. 54.

58. Rodríguez Expósito, "La primera secretaria de sanidad," p. 16.

59. Speech of Pedro Albarrán, reproduced in Ibid., pp. 53-55.

60. Speech of Fernando Méndez Capote, reproduced in Rodríguez Expósito, "La primera secretaria de sanidad," p. 52.

61. Circular to local sanitary officers, by Carlos J. Finlay, Chief of Sanitation, August 28, 1907, reproduced in Rodríguez Expósito, "La primera secretaria de sanidad," pp. 23-24.

62. César Rodríguez Expósito, *Dr. Juan Guiteras* (Havana: Editorial Cubanicán, 1947) p. 165. From a family of political progressives, Juan's second cousin (grandson to his father's brother) was Antonio Guiteras, the forceful and impatient revolutionary of the 1930s.

63. The Centro Asturiano was not the first association to be established, but it easily became the largest. Founded in 1885 by a breakaway faction of the Sociedad Asturiana de Beneficiencia, the center set out from the beginning to provide social, educational, and medical services for its members; to this end, contracts were arranged with one physician, three pharmacies, and with the "three best hospitals of the period, the Quinta del Rey, La Benéfica, and La Integridad Nacional." Leadership (and capital for expansion) came from the wealthiest Spanish Asturians. The first president (Don Diego González del Valle) was from a distinguished family and the second and third were, respectively, a rich tobacco manufacturer and a wealthy banker. In 1895 the society began the erection of its own clinic-hospital, the Quinta Covadonga, on the Havana estate of the second president. As if in competition with improvements in Mercedes hospital, a surgical amphitheater and other facilities were added in 1900. In good measure, the Centros Sociales *were* the

governments of the Spanish sector after independence, with great sums spent on internal political campaigns. The growth of the Centro Asturiano appears as follows:

Table 4.3
Growth of the Centro Asturiano, 1886-1945

Year	Patients Assisted in Clinics	Number of Members	Number of Students
1886	246	2,550	749
1887	1,145	2,950	
1901	5,000	10,975	
1905	12,621	25,004	
1910	—	29,000	2,984
1911	8,526	22,000	4,000
1914		37,281	
1920		47,603	
1928		60,278	
1933		30,000	
1945		40,000	

These statistics include new "delegations" in Pinar del Río, Marianao, Regla, Guanabacoa, and Tampa, Florida in 1900, with a total of 33 delegations in 1905. 1893 was marked by the purchase of the Casino Español, "the finest building in Havana;" women were admitted to classes in 1910; and 1924 saw the inauguration of a two million dollar facility and equal membership status for women. See Joseph F. Thorning, "Social Medicine in Cuba," *The Americas*, 1 (April 1945) 4: 440-55.

5
The Third Medical Revolution, 1925-1945

The third revolution in Cuban medicine was an *organizational* revolution in the sense that it resolved the burning questions of what kinds of organizations would dispense medical services in presocialist Cuba and who would control them. Four categories of organizations competed for hegemony: (1) a small number of very large prepaid medical plans that were directed by the oldest ethnic or regional associations of the Spanish;[1] (2) a large and growing number of relatively small, private or cooperative, prepaid medical plans whose origin was not directly related to the problems of new immigrants; (3) public assistance for the poor; and (4) private fee-for-service practice in various settings — office, private clinic, or, significantly, in some combination with the aforesaid categories. The conflicts and antagonisms among the four partially overlapping sectors of practitioners and patients manifested themselves most visibly in the history of the Cuban Medical Federation (FMC). On a sidestage in this drama appear, on the one hand, the alternately moderating and intervening Cuban government and, on the other hand, the shifting role of the university.[2] The background, of course, is formed by certain rather well-known economic, demographic, and political developments.

North American intervention and popular disenchantment with early republican governments left the nation's idealism estranged from public office, while the sugar economy seemed to genuflect independently before the world market. The grand boom and bust of 1925-1929-1933 coincided with the rise and fall of the dictator Gerardo Machado, a period of turmoil which was finally forced into an unsatisfying peace by World War II.

The economy and psychology of boom and bust left their mark on the health system, if only because the instability which affected the lives of consumers of health services also introduced instability into the income that could be derived from entrepreneurial medical practice. While physicians were naturally stimulated to establish private office locations conveniently near Havana's newest wealthy suburban expansion, physicians were also motivated to develop clinics which employed prepayment schemes. Prepaid clinic practice offered a degree of income stability and effective competition with the large Spanish plans. In the discussion which follows, the conflicts between physicians and prepayment plans (and among the plans themselves) occupy a central position. Unlike the course of similar conflicts in other countries, the dissatisfactions of physicians served less to limit the role of the clinic prepayment mechanism than to diversify it. The natural response of disgruntled partners, competing private physicians and physician employees was less to retreat into private offices than to regroup and establish new plans.

The Spanish ethnic associations play a role in Cuban medical conflicts and warrant yet another word of introduction. The *centros regionales* figured in the history of Cuban medicine not only because they directed key parts of urban medical care but also for the simple reason that they were prominent organizations in Cuban society. They were, however, prominent in different ways. In the midst of economic instability, the programs of the ethnic associations provided many with a valuable measure of social security; but in the smoldering postindependence years, the *centros* also appeared as disguised fortresses of the old colony; and in an emerging period of class conscious radicalism, the Spanish social clubs seemed to function as bastions of petit bourgeois conservatism. It is thus difficult in any analysis of later conflicts to isolate purely professional or occupational matters from other lines of conflict (ethnicity, nationalism, class) which overlay one another in Cuban society and which variously involved both the medical profession and the ethnic associations.

A proper history of ethnic associations in Cuba (which awaits its author) would examine the role of anarcho-syndicalism in the early organizational impulse of the associations, their capture by political conservatism, and gradual diminution of ethnic identification after the Second World War. The ethnic societies dominated much of early twentieth-century metropolitan social life. When, for example, the Centro Asturiano held elections for officers (in this mini-government of the ethnic community) everyone in Havana knew about it. Newspapers, streets, and sidewalks were filled with the slogans and exhortations of the candidates and their tightly-organized political factions. This highly visible mode of organization and activism left its stamp on the larger society and influenced, I believe, the decisively organizational bent of Cuban medicine and the political mold of its federation. This influence, however imprecise, was both direct, in the actual control by ethnic associations over certain medical institutions, and indirect, in providing models of activism and in providing a focus of conflict for medical unity.

CUBAN MEDICAL FEDERATION

The history of the Cuban Medical Federation (FMC), often regarded by Cuban physicians as the struggle of *la clase médica*, is equally the history of class and generational conflict within the profession itself, and of the eventual victory after 1940 of youthful and radical leadership.[3] It may seem strange, then, that I have previously referred to the end point of this period as one of bureaucratic entrenchment. Internally divided, the moment of victory (with increased employment security, minimum salaries, and compulsory federation of physicians) was the signal for a slide into entrenchment. This condition was sealed by the corrupt ineffectiveness of the left-liberal social democratic governments of Grau San Martín and Carlos Prío,[4] the very governments which one might have expected to have opened new horizons to the progressives who led the FMC. This period, which might be interpreted as revealing some of the constraints to reform under left-liberal governments, was followed by the pall cast over Cuban institutions by the Batista tyranny.

Foundation and Early Fragmentation

In 1929, four years after the formation of the Cuban Medical Federation, the first internal political parties took form. One group, known as Renovación, was composed mainly of younger physicians who did not work for mutualist programs; their chief concern was the extraordinary increase in "pseudo-mutualisms."[5] Renovistas also called for greater freedom for private practice, and at the same time, higher wages and better university training. The other principal faction, Unión Federativa, consisted of physicians who predominantly gave services to large mutualist programs. Renovación was led by Alberto Recio y Forns,[6] a protegé of Juan Guiteras and from one of Havana's oldest families. In concert with Ángel Arturo Aballí,[7] Recio and a group of collaborators at the Mercedes Hospital had provided the impulse to take over the languid Colegio Médico de Cuba and form the Medical Federation. One would suppose that Recio's faction appealed to the predominant interests of the profession, for the 1925 call for the founding convention had gathered two thousand enthusiastic physicians from all parts of the island. The working meetings covered relations with the regional centers, relations with the government, immoral exercise of the profession, relations between physicians, and professional honoraria.[8]

The First National Convention on Mutualism, sponsored by the FMC in the wake of their first strike from 1927 to 1928 against the Centro Gallego called for: prohibition against mutualist services for well-to-do patients, suppression of "industrialism", and provision of mutualist services to members only and not to pensioners. The demands reflected the irritation experienced by physicians when desirable private clients took advantage of the inexpensive group prepayment mechanism and thus further restricted the field for lucrative independent and fee-for-service practice. "Industrialism" was a vague reference to the increased efficiency of the large hospital centers and the tendency for physicians to work as mere wage-laborers. But the proposed restrictions on pensioners suggests a note of desparation in the quest for private patients. These bases for mutualism were nominally accepted by some mutualities, but not by the Centro Gallego. For the next fifteen or more years, the dilemma of mutualism and antagonism with the regional centers would be on the FMC agenda.

Related within the spirit of the times to the birth of the FMC was the formation, also in 1925, of the Cuban Communist Party and the Cuban Confederation of Workers.

Machado and Union Federativa

The link to government was established from the beginning. The new and apparently able president Gerardo Machado, anticipating an important event, made appearances at the founding convention of the FMC and again at the Convention on Mutualism in 1928, always surrounded by a group of medical supporters. Every meeting of the FMC gave its formal praise and support to Machado until 1929, when four physicians resigned in protest. On the way toward arbitrary rule, Machado had managed a temporary solution to the conflict with the Centro Gallego, and the FMC readmitted expelled strikebreakers to the medical fold.[9] But sensing his true interests, Machado cultivated even stronger links to the Spanish business colony, which dominated the ethnic associations. The most powerful man in Machado's administration, Thomas concludes, was Viriato Gutiérrez, the son-in-law and heir of Laureano Falla Gutiérrez, the largest Spanish sugar mill owner in Cuba.[10]

The federation fell more strongly into the hands of dictator Machado when, in 1929, Renovación lost the National Assembly elections to Unión Federativa, led by Francisco María (Panchón) Fernández,[11] Machado's secretary of sanitation and charities. By 1930, there were greater tensions as the economy slumped and suppression of dissent grew more violent, even to the point of outraging the professional and middle classes. Labor leaders and Spanish anarchists were exiled, imprisoned or murdered. Four students were dropped to the sharks. Student and labor leader Julio Antonio Mella was assassinated by Machado's agents in Mexico City, followed by the death of the medical student Rafael Trejo. Renewed protests led to the closing of the university and some fifty rebellious professors were fired.[12] Members of the Marxist oriented Ala Izquierda Estudiantil were imprisoned, including the medical students, Gustavo Aldereguía, Alejandro Vergara, Rodríguez Pintado, a certain Carreras, and others, along with some professors. Alongside such distinguished thinkers as Raúl Roa (later president of the Social Science Faculty and, with the socialist revolution, Foreign Minister of Cuba), prison became a university for Marxist revolutionaries.

With such matters in the minds and conversations of physicians, especially in the Colegio Médico de la Habana,[13] the conservative Francisco Maria Fernández and Ricardo Núñez Portuondo editorialized in the *Tribuna Médica* (the official organ of the FMC): "The legitimate right of physicians to freely occupy their place in the columns of different opinions, according to their own criteria and personal feelings was endangering, . . . by the propagation of passionate exhortations of an ideological nature external to our problems, the fraternal march of the Federation."[14]

The anticipated split within the FMC was avoided by compromises at the December 1930 meeting held in Santa Clara and reflecting this compromise, successful efforts were made to improve the treatment of medical prisoners held by Machado. A delegation from Mayarí, Oriente Province, offered a resolution in favor of Workers' Accident Insurance, reflecting the presence of a large sugar mill in that town. A charity fund was established for poor physicians, and Dr. Ortiz Cano, indicating another trend of the times, introduced a resolution on "Specialties and Post Graduate School." Aballí, as usual, spoke in favor of increased professional freedoms and private practice.

Increasing Conflict and Medical Insurgency

The years 1931 and 1932 saw increased conflicts, not all of them approved or directed, by the FMC, especially with La Bondad and La Balear and strikes against the Centro Castellano, the Centro Canario, and the Colonia Español of Santa Clara. Two important principles were adopted by the FMC in these years: the Second Convention on Mutualism in 1931 issued an explicit condemnation of multiple position holding by physicians, and the FMC National Assembly of 1932 chose to eliminate the five-year waiting period between graduation from medical school and admission to the FMC. The latter resolution forbode a flood of new members from a turbulent university, who were yet unmellowed by five years of medical practice. The resolution on multiple positions was stated in the strongest possible terms, although evidently without any means of enforcement: "*That no motive may justify as moral or scientific the hoarding of various positions in different public or private services.*"[15] (The quote appears in bold face type, underlined, in the source cited.) Conflicts with mutualism extended to Cienfuegos, Camagüey, Santiago, Matanzas, and Unión de Reyes in the last year of the Machado tyranny, and the FMC demanded power to oversee the admission of members to mutualist plans. Reflecting the entrance of many young members into the FMC, Renovación split into two new parties: Reformista, led by Alfredo Antonetti Vivar, and the Ala Izquierda led by Gustavo Aldereguía. Unión Federativa continued, under attack, and a new FMC party AFPEL (Federated Group for Free Practice), the most direct expression of U.S. medicine, was led by Félix Lancís.

In 1932, amid an atmosphere of daily murders, the medical crisis came to a head immediately before the fall of Machado with the declaration of a general strike against the regional centers. This was only one of several strikes in the service sector that were occurring at the time. Theoretically strengthening the position of the FMC, the weak, but modestly revolutionary, new government of Grau San Martín decreed the Obligatory Federation of Physicians. In response, the powerful Spanish colony showed its teeth: "the Spanish societies organized a monstrous demonstration which ran through the principal streets and filed past the First Magistrate of the Nation," prompting President Grau to subject the problems to further study. (The fall of Machado also precipitated the resignation of some FMC executives, including its president.) Physicians responded with a protest at the Spanish embassy and, with a great deal of general anti-Spanish feeling in the air, including anti-Spanish riots, the December National Assembly of the FMC elected to extend the general strike to all of the principal groups in Cuba.[16] An accord was finally reached in January 1934, with a government assurance, which proved hollow, of a minimum wage and the submission of other strike disputes to arbitration by the International Labor Office (ILO) under the League of Nations. The ILO study that was consequently prepared provides essential data on medical organization of the time.

But the settlement was too slow to avert demonstrations, in which the young physician José Elías Borges was killed. Borges, who thus became the martyr of the combative medical federation, was one of many Cuban university youths who, when forced into exile, increasingly chose France or Mexico before the United States. In France, Borges had found Marxist friends and returned to Cuba with an internationalist's bent toward revolution. He was not an anarchist, as Hugh Thomas has said, but was rather a member of the Communist Party, one of some thirty Havana physicians who were then carrying the red card.[17] Hugh Thomas describes the period thus:

> Revolutionary demands existed on all sides; all parties declared themselves to be revolutionary, and protests continued. In February 30,000 tobacco workers struck. Various strikes continued in the sugar mills [with workers in possession of some 40 mills under a call from the C.P. to form a Red Army], and even doctors and nurses struck against Spanish private medical schemes, with extraordinary scenes at hospitals: patients were turned away, while doctors were seen stomping up and down the Prado singing the *International*. No death certificates were given and coffins piled up. One doctor was shot and buried in a red flag. Bombs exploded throughout the island . . .[18]

Repression by the Counterrevolution

The Grau regime was unable to restore order and consolidate power chiefly because the U.S. refused to recognize his government. Thus, Col. Fulgencio Batista moved to become the strong man behind the acceptable new president, Carlos Mendieta.[19] One of his first actions was to suspend the decree of compulsory professional federation, thus reversing the advance of physicians. Protesting, the FMC expelled Santiago Verdega, Director of Sanitation, who promulgated the unpopular order. Improved wages and conditions were won, however, in eleven government-related institutions including hospitals, dispensaries, and institutes.

The next year the FMC formulated new demands. They called for a minimum wage of one hundred dollars for all municipal sanitation directors, and demanded that pensioners be excluded from hospitals wherever private clinics existed. When physicians struck the municipal services of Havana in 1935, police moved to occupy dispensaries. Faced with insurgency and violence, Batista's police took over the university and its hospital, Calixto García. A medical strike further resulted in massive suppression of physicians. Sympathizers of the FMC were fired in all government-related institutions. Under Batista's plan for his new army, a quasi-fascist Military Medical Reserve was formed, forcing all but notorious radicals into service and giving them civilian posts. On March 19, 1935, the FMC was declared illegal and its offices destroyed. The Ley Docente of the rebellious puppet president, Miguel Mariano Gómez[20] offered, however, a new compromise and in 1938 the FMC reappeared with a comprehensive platform calling for pharmaceutical controls, workers' accident protection, a minimum wage scale for physicians, prohibition on multiple positions, institutionalization of the sanitary career, improved hospitals, school health, sanitary provisions for the poor, government support against professional intrusion, a physicians' retirement plan, and (again) limitations on the *centros regionales*.[21]

In the interim, from 1936 to 1937, the underground expression of the Medical Federation had appeared disguised as another medical journal, *Medicina de Hoy*, and was influenced, it seems, by members of the Ala Izquierda such as Federico Sotolongo, one of several who demonstrated that old aristrocratic families could wear revolutionary colors. An editorial of 1936 called for the creation of the sanitary career:

In Cuba . . ., the medical positions in the sanitary service are obtained without having . . . elementary notion of . . . the obligations that should be carried out and that are realized by any true sanitarian.

Thus . . . the fellows [who occupy sanitary posts] generally deprecate their obligations to society, ganging together and serving the political group that makes use of them.[22]

Thus, the article continues, sanitary work cannot develop as a specialty, which would require improved salaries and the separation of hiring and firing from political influence.

Acción Inmediata

Although the direction of the reopened FMC seems to have reflected the thinking of the Ala Izquierda, as "respectable" physicians reincorporated, the FMC, nonetheless remained under the control of the Unión Federativa. But a flood of new physicians, formed by years of university and national strife entered the FMC and inaugurated a new medical party known as Acción Inmediata. Under leadership of the class of 1937 and, later, the class of 1940,[23] the new medical party was apparently allied with older leaders of the Ala Izquierda. In a process of polarization, the highly disciplined propaganda and political work within the FMC of Acción Inmediata unified their opposition into yet another party, the Ortodoxos (not directly connected, I think, to the national political party of the same name) led by José Bisbé. But the unity behind the Ortodoxos was incomplete, drawing support to a small core of men around Bisbé from old followers of Unión Federativa and Reformista, the conservative wing of the old Renovación. A generational element was clearly involved. Acción Inmediata directed propaganda and organizing efforts at university students, causing each new class of graduates to fall into the ranks of the insurgent faction. Eventual victory seemed certain. The menace of the youthful party created the most decisive cleavage ever to exist within the FMC. The first demand on the extensive 1938 platform of Acción Inmediata was "Puesto único y sueldo mínimo!" ("Single post and minimum wage!") Although this demand was the cutting edge of conflict in the FMC, the other demands are interesting to note, for they are an indication of the combination of interests served and the development of a significant philosophy of social medicine. Moreover, most of the demands were realized in one form or another in the next few years.[24] Many of the demands of the FMC were included in the Constitution of 1940, indicating the considerable power of physicians and other professional groups (linked in a Confederation of University Professions) in the framing of the liberal constitution.

The brief consensus which launched the Constitution of 1940, followed by the constitutional presidencies of Batista (1940), Grau San Martín (1945), and Carlos Prío (1950), strengthened the position of the FMC. In the consensus of 1940, a general agreement between FMC belligerents and the *centros regionales* and other mutualities was reached, and FMC and non-FMC physicians were rehired, with the clinching proviso that all new physicians would be federated. One physician settled for back pay, but loudly protested when he was refused the right to name his successor, an interesting incident which suggests a common practice.[25] The progressives within the FMC inspired the formation of a commission on parasitism and infant and neonatal mortality, and also a tax of 2 percent on physicians' income exceeding one hundred dollars per month. It seems difficult to believe that the latter measure could have been carried out.

Resistance to vehement agitation of Acción Inmediata for implementation of the FMC proscription of multiple positions provided for an extraordinary National Assembly in 1940. Over angry protests of Acción Inmediata, Ortodoxo leaders José Bisbé and Laudelindo González proposed that attempts to implement the regulation should be dropped until minimum wage, compulsory federation, and professional immobility were won. (The Constitution of 1940 was only slowly and never completely implemented in actual legislation.) The Ortodoxo amendment passed by a vote of 110 to 90. Angrily, the progressive young Catholic, Juan Antonio Rubio Padillo, hinted at the demise of the federation: "There is nothing to discuss from now on . . . the matter sleeps in a tomb that has been tightly nailed, tightly with roses." Bisbé replied, "What one must do is to come here with a majority and not to make lamentations when you don't have the medical majority." President Batista promptly and graciously decreed that university professors could occupy more than one post in his government.[26]

Defeat of the Old Guard

But Acción Inmediata was gaining the majority. In 1941, they won the leadership of the Havana Medical College, a victory that was temporarily reversed in 1942 when over one thousand combative physicians turned out for the annual meeting. In 1942, the leadership of the FMC fell to Acción Inmediata and, in 1943, the majority in the Havana Medical College, with more than one thousand members, turned in the same direction.

In turning over power, the previous leadership set a bad example. Anticipating defeat and smarting under sharpened criticism, leading members of the Executive Committee resigned, *before* the new election, followed after the election by the resignation of the entire office staff. Indeed, it sounded like momentous occasion of state. On inauguration as president of the FMC, Luis Antonio de la Cruz Muñoz was eloquent: "Victory does not make us proud for we regard it as a dangerous illusion, inasmuch as life is struggle and constant progression and one does not triumph thus, completely never; nor do we fear failure for we know that the failure of some will support the rectified action of others."[27]

Action did seem to follow immediately. Single post, $100 minimum monthly salary, and a physicians' retirement plan were decreed by Batista's government in 1943. Compulsory federation was decreed in 1944. In addition to government acquiescence to FMC objectives, the new FMC organized the First Cuban Conference on Nutrition, an incredible assembly of more than fifty organizations, from the Anti-Imperialist League of the

Communists to the United Fruit Company, an assembly possible only in the middle of war (World War II), for which physicians were busily organizing sanitary preparations. The conference was extremely successful, creating a National Milk Institute, a Livestock Directory, and suggesting other constructive proposals. Responding to the political sophistication of the times, the Womens' Section of Acción Inmediata was established in 1943, with ten or more activists dedicated especially to problems of women physicians, most of them recent graduates of the university. By 1945, there were only thirty women among the one thousand Havana physicians.[28]

STRUCTURE OF HEALTH SERVICES

To understand why the conflict among physicians suddenly took such proportions, one must remember that while new members were added to the profession, the sharp and popular conflicts with the Spanish centers and with Machado and Mendieta-Batista had united many physicians, while other serious points of difference had been swept aside. Important sources of conflict were sidestepped simply by proclaiming all views, without being put to the test of implementation. A more complete picture of the structure of medical practice is necessary.

Distribution of Health Resources

The medical situation was, to begin with, completely different in Havana from what it was in the rest of Cuba. The contrast appears in Tables 5.1 and 5.2.

Clearly, the major *objective* contradiction in medical care in the 1920s and 1930s, indeed in the whole presocialist period, lay in the disparity between urban and rural health care; but this contradiction was inadequately expressed by mobilized constituencies, particularly among physicians. Thus, the tempestuous history of the medical federation is primarily an expression of the contradictions within the urban sphere of medical practice. (Some exceptions are worthy of note, but in order to limit redundancy I will defer discussion of rural health care to another section which discusses the rural health services established in 1959.) Granting even that some important national services should be located in the capital, the concentration of personnel and services was extreme. Almost half of all physicians and more than half of all hospital beds were in Havana. The 1934 report by the International Labor Office immediately concluded: "The plethora of physicians is evident and would without doubt be enough by itself to make the situation difficult for Havana physicians."[29] Yet the extreme concentration becomes even more pronounced when the working context of urban physicians is broken down. The same report provides the

Table 5.1
Physicians in Provinces and in the
City of Havana, 1934*

Province	Population	Rural Physicians**	Total Physicians	Inhabitants per Physician
Pinar del Rio	343,820	28	130	2,645
Havana (Interior)	443,000	32	216	2,050
Matanzas	337,119	15	164	2,056
Santa Clara	815,412	62	317	2,572
Camagüey	408,076	51	175	2,332
Oriente	1,072,757	80	340	3,155
Totals (Interior)	3,420,184	268	1,342	2,250
Havana (City)	542,500	—	1,200	450
Totals (Cuba)	3,962,684	268	2,542	1,559

*Data are derived from Cyrille Dechamp and Moisés Poblete Troncoso, *El problema médico y la asistencia mutualista en Cuba*, a report of the International Labor Office, Havana, 1934, pp. 28-29.

**No definition, unfortunately, is given.

Table 5.2
National and Municipal Hospitals, 1934

Province	Number of Hospitals	Number of Physicians	Number of Beds	Population	Inhabitants per Bed
Pinar del Rio	3	6	380	343,820	2,642
Havana (Interior)**	4	11	115	443,000	3,900
Matanzas	5	19	329	337,119	1,025
Santa Clara	7	19	589	815,412	1,042
Camagüey	2	6	222	408,076	1,793
Oriente	9	18	454	1,072,757	2,363
Totals (Interior)	30	69	2,089	3,420,184	1,700
Havana (City)	6	183	3,014	542,500	180
Totals (Cuba)	36	252	5,103	3,962,684	776

*Data are derived from Cyrille Dechamp and Moisés Poblete Troncoso, *El problema médico y la asistencia mutualista en Cuba*, a report of the International Labor Office, Havana, 1934, pp. 28-29.

essential data. (See Table 5.3.) Although the estimates used here were probably derived from the parties involved and might be biased; they no doubt represent the general patterns of practice.

Table 5.3
Four Sectors of Services in Havana, 1934 *

	Centros Regionales, Old Mutualism	New Mutualism	Public Assistance	Private
Number of people covered	100,000 (18% of Havana's population)	107,000 (20% of Havana's population)	198,500 (36% of Havana's population)	136,500 (25% of Havana's population)
Number of separate institutions	Few: 3 accounted for 75% and 4 accounted for 90% of members	Many: 32 groups with 500 to 15,000 members	Two large hospitals (Mercedes & Calixto Garcia) and several small institutions	Several non-mutualist private clinics, one small elite general hospital
Number of beds	Many: 3,300 in 3 mutualities (1 per 23 members)	Few: small hospital-clinics	3,000 (1 per 67 "Poor" or 1 per 112 persons not in mutualism)	Few
Physicians	75	557	183	385 unattached physicians and sanitary officials
Number of members per physician	1,330	194	1,085	355
Beds per physician	44 +	Very small number	16	undetermined
Composition of members	Predominantly Spanish. Small merchants, artisans, some workers	Cuban middle class, stable workers, professionals	Predominantly black and mulatto underclass (1/3 of total population)	Unstable workers, some of every class, especially the rich
Services provided	Hospitalization, dispensary services in some but not all. Charges: $2/month	Home care at $1/month Some: hospitalization and dispensary at $2 per month	Free services for hospitalization only	Variable; home and office visits

*Data are adapted from Cyrille Dechamp and Moisés Poblete Troncoso, *El problema médico y la asistencia mutualista en Cuba*, a report of the International Labor Office, Havana, 1934.

Table 5.4*
Four Sectors of Services in the Interior, 1934

	Centros Regionales, Old Mutualism	New Mutualism	Public Assistance	Private
Salaries of physicians	Specialist part time, $125/month; generalist full time, $150; intern, $100; Chief of services: $160	Generalist full time, $60-$80/month	Generalist full time, $87/month	Income extremely variable
Number of people covered	35,000-40,000 in both kinds of mutualism, mostly delegations of Havana Centros Regionales	See Appendix	3,552,200 in both categories	
Number of physicians	undetermined	undetermined	267 (69 in hospitals)	1,343
Number of units	8	few	30 hospitals, average bed size of 67, only a few are larger	
Number of beds	undetermined	undetermined	2,089 (1/1700 pop.)	

*Data are derived from Dechamp and Troncoso, *El problema médico y la asistencia médica mutualista en Cuba*, Havana, 1934.
Excluded from consideration here are 2,610 beds of the Mazorra National Psychiatric Hospital (still known as the Asylum for the Aged Slaves).

Old and New Mutualism

Perhaps 36 percent of Havana's population were covered under some form of "mutualism," to use the term somewhat loosely, which employed over half of all physicians and owned more than half of Havana's beds. But mutualism was of two general types, what I shall call (with some inaccuracy) "old" and "new." "Old mutualism" was developed, roughly, in the 1880s, oriented toward the problems of Spanish immigrants and organized by Spanish ethnic and commercial associations. For reasons that I have already suggested, these medical programs grew rapidly after 1902 when the conditions of the new republic brought an avalanche of immigration from declining Spain. Two hundred thousand arrived between 1902 and 1910[30] with a rate of some 30,000 per year between 1914 and 1918 and 10,000 per year thereafter until about 1925.[31]

Into the category of "new mutualism" are classed the small mutualist programs which sprang up after around 1905, especially after 1920, and which received a new burst of growth in the period of conflict between the FMC and the *centros regionales*. "New mutualism" tended to mix the features of mutualist and nonmutualist private clinics. This tendency is explained by reference to the emerging class structure in Havana, an established tradition of small private clinics, the aggressively expansive character of old mutualism, the new capital requirements of modern medicine, and the erratic extremes of the sugar economy which simultaneously stimulated and threatened the existence of marginal clinics.[32]

Private Clinics and Pseudomutualism

Between 1902 and 1910, the population of Havana increased by more than 60,000, to 300,000, and almost doubled in geographical size. Sugar escalated toward a period of money madness from 1907 to 1912, while twenty-one new giant mills were built and Oriente was developed, again by burning forests. By 1919, the sumptuous Vedado suburb was rivalled by Miramar, and the even more extravagant Country Club section was begun. The private clinics, which sprung up amid these developments, were soon integrated into the high social life of the elite suburbs. One beckoned, for example, in an advertisement,

Señora:

We cordially invite you to visit our clinic, situated on the most aristocratic and central street of Vedado.[33]

In 1927, at the height of clinic expansion before the economic and political crisis of 1929, Emilio Roig de Leuchsenring wrote a revealing satirical sketch on social manners:

Appendicitis has come to be the true complement to the social education of the young lady . . . The work on the lower right of the ab-
domen is the rubric affixed by the surgeon to attest the aristocracy of
its bearer, a stamp more valuable than yesteryear's royal seal on let-
ters of nobility.

The corridors have the effect, for all the comings and goings, of a
ballroom in a moment when the music has stopped and the couples
pass to and fro.

Since in this large village, which is Havana, we all know one another,
friends and relatives of the different patients, we get together everyday to visit and find out "how your relative is doing" or to keep up
with the registrations and departures.

And finally, the fashionable clinics are used to such extent for child-
birth that future historians will simply publish the photographs of
the elegant clinics of our capital.[34]

In order for enterprising physicians to attract patients in the new era
and, to some degree, in order to provide quality service, one had to adver-
tise not only the names of prominent physicians, but also the names of new
equipment and procedures: "BLOOD TRANSFUSIONS," "X-RAY
ANALYSIS," "LABORATORY DIAGNOSIS," and so forth.[35] This
necessity was met by some kind of clinic, or, to raise capital, a cooperative
practice or partnership of physicians, usually dominated by a single figure,
often a university professor of exceptionally good family, or a graduate of a
North American medical school. Most often, he was a surgeon and, increasingly, one or more subspecialties were advertised.[36] The maintenance
of a basic income, as well as the struggle to entice patients away from the
centros regionales, called for an insurance plan for patients, hence,
creating the pseudomutualities. Many of these clinics were already
marginal before the crash of the sugar boom in 1920, and after this date
more clinics offered insurance programs to cushion themselves against an
adverse economy. The increases in the number of physicians, resulting
from expanded classes at the university, created larger numbers of poor
physicians, and students, who could be employed by the new mutualisms.
Marginal clinics expanded on the backs of marginal physicians. The directors or owners of such clinics sought to maintain a reasonable salary or a
return on capital investment; the latter varied a great deal and was often
quite small. If the clinic became famous (and there was much overt advertising, unheard of in sedate North American practice), the clinic's leading
physicians would become rich, acquiring a private practice. The bulk of
new mutualities were, of course, in the better suburbs, while the *centros
regionales* were located in older sections of the city. Since the regional
centers increasingly restricted outpatient services, the new mutualist
programs were made more attractive by offering home visits.[37]

The Principal Contradiction within Mutualism

While hospital beds were concentrated in old mutualism, physicians came to be concentrated in the new. The social contradiction was obvious.

Under old mutualism, hospital beds were consistently underutilized, with hardly one-third of the beds occupied in 1934 by patients with acute medical conditions.[38] But old mutualism was efficient, perhaps to the point of declining quality, in the use of physicians, with 75 physicians for 100,000 members, (see Table 5.2), mostly in four or five principal centers. New mutualism was highly inefficient, employing some 557 physicians in 32 groups with a combined total of no more than 107,000 members. This category of groups had, on the whole, extremely limited facilities; while a jealously regarded elite of larger and longer established groups, in the category of new mutualism, were known for their sophisticated clinics and services to wealthy patients.

While some of the first conflicts in the FMC appeared to be between physicians within mutualism and those outside of mutualism, the first effective alliance incorporated physicians from all sectors, new mutualist, old mutualist, and nonmutualist physicians, against the *centros regionales*. Equally important, the same antagonism helped to cement bonds between entrepreneurial physicians and their employees.[39] Whether in new mutualism, private clinic, or isolated private practice, all seemed to gain from limitations on the regional centers. The predominant — and sometimes ostentatious — Spanish identity of these centers, and their generally conservative politics,[40] made them exceptional targets to unite rather disparate categories of physicians. Later, the names of early leaders of the FMC, Recio, Antonetti, and others, would appear comfortably — and ostentatiously — on the nameplates of important Havana clinics. The marginality of some of these institutions undoubtedly heightened the anxieties of conflict in the depression years that ended Machado's government and inaugurated the counterrevolution of Mendieta-Batista.

The Overlay of Private Practice

Private practice and the network of private transactions greatly modified the structure that has thus far been outlined. For private practice was by no means restricted in Havana to the 385 institutionally unattached physicians. (See Table 5.3.) Rather it was precisely the physicians who enjoyed good positions in institutions who also enjoyed greatest access to private patients, technical support, and access to hospital beds. The 385 physicians included some sanitary officials, nonpracticing physicians, and "hole-in-the-wall" physicians.[41] The specialists employed by the giant regional centers were an elite who also used the facilities for private patients. The same was also true of the smaller mutualities. What could be better than to be a private patient of Alfredo Antonetti in the Clínica Antonetti, which also had a growing mutualist program? Lesser employee-physicians simply used more humble positions as a means of building their private clientele. The overlap between private practice and mutualism led to widespread abuses, where physicians were encouraged to liberally recommend services that were not covered under mutualist programs and to recommend consultations that would return split fees. It was through such abuses that many physicians were persuaded to accept rather meager salaries and sometimes to serve without any salary at all.

Private services also existed within public institutions, and, since many new mutualities had inadequate facilities, pressures existed to make public facilities available on a privileged basis as backup facilities for mutualities and their private patients. Hospitals Mercedes and Calixto García had special beds for private patients. These were used by principal staff physicians. Such resources must have also provided important backup services for the new and poorly equipped mutualities.[42] Some departments of Calixto García kept two sets of books, one as the private clinic of its director and another as a body under the university and hospital budget.[43] Such practices may not have been as bad as it may appear, for while it did make public patients into a kind of lower class within institutions that were supposed to serve them, regular budgets were chronically insufficient (as was true of small mutualities) and the benefits of investment from private income must have served in some measure to improve or maintain the general facilities. These observations, of course, modify the meaning of figures on beds for new mutualism and public assistance, with more beds for the former, fewer for the latter, and more beds for general private practice. Powerful conflicts of interest were in any case created. All but old mutualism were favored by the expansion of public assistance, provided that it was carefully restricted to the very poor, a qualification that meant more to the entrepreneurs of marginal clinics than to anyone else.

Alternatives for the Medical Profession

The structure of contradictions within medical and hospital practice help us to understand the conflicts and perspectives that were evident in the history of the FMC. In such circumstances, what *could* have been the attitude of the FMC toward the offensive regional centers, a question the more important because the regional centers were, in some ways, the most advanced and progressive medical institutions in Cuba. The regional centers guaranteed hospital care in a time when the hospital component was becoming more and more important. Large hospitals provided the most favorable context for the development and use of specialists. One might well imagine that the integration of services was more efficient in the regional centers than in the public and university hospitals which were known for extreme decentralization into jealously isolated departments, a phenomenon which might have been reduced by a unitary administration that was somewhat removed from the interests of physicians. In short, the regional centers produced an apex of quality services and seemed to be well advanced in the technical trend of medical care. Not surprisingly, the professional salaries of old mutualism were much higher, on the average, than either new mutualism, public assistance hospitals, or sanitary posts.[44]

Almost every proposal included a call for limitations which would serve the interests of private practice, such as one proposal of the FMC that services be rendered only to persons carrying a "poor person's identification card." Dechamp and Troncoso, authors of the International Labor Office report, suggested that in the long range, the facilities of the regional centers might be integrated with the services of public assistance.[45] Such a measure would contribute to more efficient use of the old mutualist beds and resolve in part the contradiction with new mutualism. This proposal, which was not echoed by the FMC, could not be seriously proposed until greater confidence in government existed. Moreover, rationalization would not be favored by extreme proponents of private practice and would be feared by sectors of new mutualism.

One of the most imaginative and intelligent proposals came from the Ala Izquierda in 1934. Gustavo Alderguía proposed that the FMC create a national mutuality of medical assistance. Members of FMC would begin by providing medical and surgical services to all "mutualizable" (meaning not rich) members of institutions in conflict with FMC.[46] Alderguía's reasonable proposal, rejected by the Executive Committee, marks a turning point in the history of the FMC and permits one to muse over the road not taken. Private and entrepreneurial mutualist physicians naturally feared what such an organization might eventually mean and by 1934 many physicians were already trapped in the marginality of new mutualism and overextended by multiple position holding. (The commonplace holding of several positions may mean that the number of physicians employed in various institutions, especially in new mutualism, was somewhat inflated and the number of unattached physicians was probably underestimated.) In one sense, Alderguía's proposal was too late; in another sense its constituency had not yet arrived. Instead, the Executive Committee of the FMC gave its support to the formation and strengthening of medical cooperatives and other new mutualisms, "with which," comments FMC historian Fernández-Conde, "the exploitation of physician by physician was imperceptibly initiated."[47]

BUREAUCRATIC ENTRENCHMENT

In 1945, on the heels of professional immobility won in 1944,[48] Grau San Martín, elected by a thousand compromises and obligations, disarmed his factionalized support by distributing sinecures in government ministries. Five years later, Carlos Prío, elected with even greater factional problems and obligations, distributed more than 2,000 sinecures in the Ministries of Health, Labor, Interior, and Public Works.[49] Hugh Thomas assesses corruption under Grau as worse than under Batista and rivaling that of Zayas. Virtually everyone was thought to be involved and, apparently, the social stigma of graft had lost all potency, while the economy —resurrected by war—was bolstered by new sugar quotas. Pension funds of labor unions and other groups, even the government social security reserves, were stolen. Nonetheless, many good and probably sincere men were appointed to government positions. Grau named the distinguished Dr. José Antonio Presno[50] to head the Ministry of Health and Social Assistance, a position later occupied under Prío by Acción Inmediata's unblemished militant, José Antonio Rubio Padilla. Meanwhile, an ex-president of the FMC (earlier a leader with Francisco Maria Fernández, of Unión Federativa), Ricardo Núñez Portuondo, ran for president of Cuba in the elections of 1944 under the banners of the old Liberal, Republican, and Conservative parties and represented, generally, the interests of Batista. Just as Mendieta-Batista's counterrevolution had recruited the distinguished gynecologist Gustavo Cuervo Rubio[51] into the government, Batista, after overthrowing Prío in 1952, quickly recruited such notables as Alberto Recio, who served as Minister of Health.

The leftist sector in medicine, as elsewhere, fell into disarray as Grau and Prío's[52] gunmen attacked communists within labor unions and to a degree, in the FMC. The anticommunist purge, which was perhaps the most sincere aspect of Prío's government, added an intense sectarianism to other structural problems of the Ministry of Health and, one may suppose, to the functioning of the FMC, for communists were always represented in FMC leadership after 1943.

The Government Sector

As sincere and, often, Catholic social democrats, the well-intentioned men who found their way into the Grau and Prío governments were frustrated in every direction. Physicians and other professionals could not be fired from many positions without prior approval of the professional associations. It was well understood, as one ex-government official put it, what the problems of health and medical needs were among the poor and rural population, but there was simply nothing one could do. Hopes were placed, therefore, in indirect and painless forms of manipulation, most of which were never realized. Such established hierarchies could not be changed, each new government program took the form of yet another vertical structure, endlessly duplicating administrative functions.

Each new Cuban government claimed some contribution to health services and social welfare, a patchwork of activities that parallel the rocky history of the medical federation. Pushed by the earnest proposals of the medical federation, by labor unions, political parties, and the promises of electoral campaigns, a variety of health and social insurance measures were adopted and applied to restricted sectors of the population. Workers' accident insurance, retirement funds, and maternal and child health services for working women were established, along with special services for specialized disease categories — tuberculosis, leprosy, and venereal disease. Under Batista's early military plans for rural Cuba, an institute for rural medicine was formed.

But while government-supported programs in public health expanded, particularly after 1933 and again after 1945, the structure of activities directly controlled by the Ministerio de Salubridad y Asistencia Social did not change greatly. By the end of the presocialist period, the ministry directed thirty small hospitals and dispensaries of various kinds in all of Cuba. But five tuberculosis hospitals and twenty-eight dispensaries were directed by the autonomous Consejo Nacional de Tuberculosis. Similar facilities for leprosy, venereal disease, and certain dermatoses were administered by the Patronato para la Lepra y Enfermedades Cutáneas y Venéreas. The same was true of the rather limited Instituto Técnico de Salubridad Rural. The Organización Nacional de Dispensarios Infantiles (ONDI) directed four hospitals and thirty-two dispensaries; the Organización Nacional de Recuperación de Inválidos (ONRI) and the Seguro de Maternidad had five hospitals. Finally, in the largest municipalities, like Havana and Santiago, there were municipal facilities, a small number of hospitals, and a larger number of dispensaries. The Mazorra Hospital for the Insane, with more than three thousand inmates, was, again, a separate administration. And the three university hospitals, with 1,700 beds in 1959, were totally independent. Local sanitary boards were rudimentary, except in metropolitan areas.[53]

Similar observations apply to medical education. The technical standards of medical instruction were thought to have declined in the inefficient organization of autonomous departmental hierarchies, but there was no way to impose reform on the university. The professors of the university were being courted on every side and hence could not be moved. Accordingly, a plan was proposed to develop a rival medical school, connected to a prestigious North American university such as Harvard, to simultaneously serve as its adjunct school of tropical medicine. The plan, which would have taken several years of political stability to accomplish, should be considered as a manifestation of the bankruptcy of alternatives. Interviews with many Cuban physicians verify that there were simply no other practical plans or ideas for resolving the glaring contradictions in the Cuban health system.

Meanwhile, professional protection of immobility rights and compulsory federation, seemed simply to return the system to the colonial era.

Once again, although the practice had evidently continued throughout the years, physicians clung tenaciously to several positions, sometimes with fraudulent names, and rented them out when the need arose to subordinate physicians. At one extreme of absurdity, student interns in hospitals would hold their positions for years.

Mutualism and the Centro Benéfico de los Trabajadores de Cuba

When such circumstances were combined with an overall demographic and economic expansion (although not one which favored the latter over the former), it is understandable that the trends and problems earlier described simply blossomed in the third postrevolutionary period. New mutualism, now not at all new, more successfully competed with the old mutualism of the regional centers. The mutualist clinic owned by Alfredo Antonetti, the old leader of the medical faction "Renovación," assisted by an ample family of physicians, became one of the most prestigious.[54] Still another element of mutualist diversity was added in 1938, when, the communist-led Transport Workers Union inaugurated a prepaid clinic and health plan for its members — the Centro Benéfico y Jurídico de los Trabajadores de La Habana. Dramatically successful after the first difficult five years, the Centro Benéfico offered its plan to other workers in Havana and later to workers in other cities. By 1959, the plan enrolled some 25,000 subscribers.

The uniqueness of one feature of the Centro Benéfico tells more about mutualism in general than it does about the Centro itself: *the Centro Benéfico was the only mutualist clinic which served a substantial number of nonwhite Cubans and served them without discrimination or segregation.* Ethnic centers and prestigious clinics barred nonwhites from entrance, and nowhere, except in parts of the public sector and in the Centro Benéfico, were nonwhite patients given beds adjacent to whites. This implicit racism was so widely practiced and taken for granted that it was not until I examined the Centro Benéfico in detail that I learned about the prevailing racial discrimination in the rest of mutualism. This racism was otherwise disguised by the "ethnic" character of old mutualism and also by the coincidence that the nonwhite population tended also to belong to the poorer one-half of Havana which could not easily afford the mutualist prepayment. The reality was, however, a rather consistent practice of segregation or exclusion throughout the private clinic and mutualist sector.

Against substantial resistence from the local medical associations in other cities, the Centro Benéfico followed the pattern set by other mutualist plans and set up "delegations" in interior cities. Meanwhile, as it grew and changed its name to the Centro Benéfico y Jurídico de los Trabajadores de *Cuba*, the Centro came to enjoy a reputation for medical excellence and organizational innovation. It created medical scholarships, published a journal, pioneered a team approach to care, and developed a self-consciously preventive approach to medicine.[55]

How then to evaluate mutualism, in all its diversity, at the end of the presocialist era? Simple quantitative evaluation reveals its strengths: in 1933 under the weight of severe economic depression, about one-third of Havana's population had been covered in some way by mutualism, a fraction which was now approaching one-half in 1958, with some 350,000 in other cities. In 1952, mutualism absorbed almost forty percent of all direct consumer expenditures for health care.[56] As at the end of the preceding revolutionary period, mutualism again appeared to be the principal arena of institutional development in health care. This is surely true also in qualitative terms, if only in reference to the services of the Centro Benéfico y Jurídico de los Trabajadores de Cuba.

But mutualism, by its urban concentration and its ability to include many marginal physicians and marginal institutions, continued to have an effect that was important throughout the period: mutualism served as an urban magnet to marginal physicians who might otherwise have followed equally marginal careers in rural communities. The subscribers of mutualism, the better employed and commercial middle classes, were thereby protected from the expense of private care (fee-for-service), on the one hand, and the inadequacies of public facilities, which were nominally free, on the other. Quite another consequence, however, of mutualism is that it lay a basis for a collective orientation to medical work and for the eventual surppression of private practice under socialism. For while mutualism may have been *mis*developed, private practice remained, by the standards of comparable societies, *under*developed.

Some would also add, I am sure, that mutualism diluted public support for the government sector. At first glance, this seems to be definitely true in the Cuban case; but it is also a beguiling simplification of underlying assumptions and complex theoretical considerations. What is certain is that the third revolution in medical care preempted private practice and launched elements of the philosophy of social medicine in the organization of clinical practice and the ideology of the medical profession. If the ideas bore insufficient fruit, it was the fault more of the public contradictions of the society than of any private cynicism of individuals.

Given a history of often valiant good intentions, it was not altogether unreasonable that at the outset of the revolution in 1959, many of the frustrated former members of Accion Inmediata should envision a simple return to the status quo of 1945 or to the nostalgic consensus of 1940, only this time under honest government. Such hopeful retrogression was soon preempted by the militant and socialist character of the snowballing Cuban Revolution, of which the contemporary, or fourth, medical revolution became an integral part. There were also physicians who in the course of medical and political struggles from 1925 to 1945 had come to regard socialism as a means of implementing the practical objectives of social medicine. Inasmuch as the new revolution would not be compromised with professional immobility and strict autonomy of the university and its professions, only such physicians could easily sacrifice the professional privileges that had been won and consolidated in the bureaucratic entrenchment of the third medical revolution.

NOTES

1. Ethnic and regional are roughly equivalent since the ethnicity is derived from historical difference between the different regions of Spain: Galicia, Asturias, Andalusia, the Canary Islands, Castille, and so forth. While an ethnic medical plan was organized by Afro-Cubans, it probably numbered no more than 1,000 members. The counterpoint to Spanish immigration, the introduction of 150,000 poverty-stricken black workers from neighboring Haiti and Jamaica further divided the nonwhite population. See Thomas, p. 524.

2. The basic reforms of the university favored medical students after 1900. In 1901-02, 266 of all 521 university students (51%) were in medicine; but in 1915-16 the figures had jumped to an unbelievable 1,036 of 1,466 or 70%! Although the beginning was prompted by greatly improved facilities and modern laboratories, the tendency after World War I turned theoretical and impractical, if only by falling behind, with a chronically inadequate budget for the number of students. See José López Sánchez, "The Teaching of Medicine in Cuba: Its Past and Present State and Prospects of Its Future Development," *Revista Finlay*, no volume indicated, (July-December 1965) 5: 63-70.

3. The main source of information for this history has been Augusto Fernández-Conde, *Biografía de la Federación Médica de Cuba* (Havana: Colegio Médico de la Habana, 1946). Fernández-Conde graduated from medical school in 1940 after several years of university and professional political involvement. Associated with a left-leaning and youthful group that eventually won elections in the FMC, he was vice-treasurer of the federation in 1946 and president of the executive committee of the Association of Graduates of 1940.

4. Social democratic in the sense that they subscribed to a variety of social welfare principles, believed in socialism as an ultimate (but faraway) goal, and were fundamentally opposed to communists, especially to any who were associated with the Soviet Union. See discussion in Thomas, pp. 650-774, especially pp. 741-44 and p. 759.

5. Pseudomutualism refers either to a private clinic which adds a prepayment program or to a clinic which pretends to be a nonprofit cooperative of physicians but in reality is an entrepreneurial venture by a partnership of physicians.

6. Alberto Recio y Forns (1885-1956) owner of a private clinic, Laboratorio Clínico del Dr. Alberto Recio, in 1936, held positions in 1929 in the following: Commission on Infectious Diseases, National Laboratory (as director), Finlay Institute, the university, and the National Commission Against Parasitism. In 1944 and again in 1952 he became Secretary of Sanitation and Hospital Assistance. See Cuba, *Directorio Professional de Medicina y Farmacia de la República de Cuba* (Havana: Rambla, Bouya and Company, 1929). See advertisement in *Tribuna Médica* 4 (May 1, 1930) 121: 10 and obituary, *Revista KUBA* 12 (1956) 7-12: 47.

7. Ángel Arturo Aballí (1880-1952) became first president of the executive committee of the new FMC. He pioneered in the specialty of pediatrics and was a professor at the University. See obituary, *Revista KUBA*, 8 (1952) 10-12: 102.

8. Fernández-Conde, p. 18.

9. Ibid., p. 41.

10. Thomas, p. 573.

11. Francisco María Fernández therefore served simultaneously as president of the Cuban League for Mental Hygiene, the Commission Against Parasitism, and the Cuban League of Social Prophylaxis (crime and delinquency prevention). A clinic for women in Calixto García also carried his name and employed some eighteen physicians and interns, along with seven nurses. (Three Cuban hospitals carried the name "General Machado.") See *Directorio Profesional*. In 1963, recalling the abuses of the past, an editorial urged physicians to "remember Panchito María Fernández." See "El X Congreso Médico-Estomatológico Nacional, *Revista Cubana de Pediatría* 35 (February 1963) 6: 1-2.

12. Thomas, pp. 591-94.

13. The Colegio Médico de La Habana continued a separate existence, apart from the FMC. Its membership, given its size, always predominated, however in the FMC.

14. Cited by Fernández-Conde, p. 43.

15. Ibid., p. 48.

16. The groups were: Centro Asturiano, Centro Gallego, Asociación de Dependientes del Comercio de La Habana, Asociación Canaria, Asociación Hijas de Galicia, Asociación Benéfica de Guantánamo, the delegations "with sanatorium" of the Centro Gallego in Santiago de Cuba and Guantánamo, and the Colonias Españolas of Matanzas, Cárdenas, Cienfuegos, Sagua la Grande, Camagüey, and Santiago de Cuba. Ibid., p. 60.

17. Daniel Alonso, personal communication, Havana, 1976.

18. Thomas, p. 691.

19. Carlos Mendieta, like Grau, and Alfredo Zayas were Cuban presidents who were trained as physicians.

20. An ambivalent figure who was elected with Batista's support but who rebelled against Batista's plan for a rural army unit of teachers and schools; he was ousted accordingly. See Thomas, pp. 704-5.

21. Fernández-Conde, p. 74. The lists of demands, of course, reflect constant grievances, not problems overcome.

22. Ramón Ibarra Pérez and Federico Sotolongo, "La Carrera Sanitaria," *Medicina de Hoy*, 1 (September 1936): 3-5.

23. The class of 1940 continued as an organized body until at least 1946. Its leadership included many active in Acción Inmediata, while many are today found in influential positions in socialized health services. Others, of course, have emigrated. See Fernández-Conde, pp. 4-5.

24. Minimum wage in 1943, compulsory federation in 1944. "Won" of course does not mean adequately enforced or without abuse.

25. A practice, one might add that dates to the sixteenth century cabildo and recognized in the university throughout most of the nineteenth and twentieth centuries. A position was regarded as personal property.

26. Fernández-Conde, pp. 105-6.

27. Ibid., p. 119.

28. Derived from Colegio Médico de La Habana, "Relación de Médicos, 1945" (no facts of publication indicated).

29. From Cyrille Dechamp and Moisés Poblete Troncoso, *El problema médico*

y la asistencia mutualista en Cuba, a report of the International Labor Office, (Havana, 1934), pp. 28-29.

30. Thomas, p. 31.

31. Ibid., p. 540.

32. The terms "old" and "new" mutualism are my own. Large versus small would be another helpful dichotomy, but I want to draw attention to plans that developed after 1915-1920 in competition or in conflict with older plans.

33. Advertisement, *Boletín Mensual de la Clínica de la Asociación de Damas de La Covadonga* 1 (July, 1934) 4: 59.

34. Roig de Leuchsenring, pp. 198-207.

35. All clinics emphasized treatment of noncontagious diseases, suggesting the closeness of the nineteenth century. Oriented to a wide category of paying patients, one advertised "rooms from $3.50 to $20.00" and another "all that is required by scientific concepts and the comfort of a first class hospital." See any number *Tribuna Médica*, 1930. In a nation of sunlight, almost every hospital had added ultraviolet equipment by 1933. See R. G. Leland, Director, Bureau of Medical Economics, American Medical Association, "The Practice of Medicine in Cuba," *The AMA Bulletin* (June 1933): 95.

36. There was yet no certification enforced for specialization. Not uncommonly a grand portrait of the owner would dominate a view of the reception room. (Not unlike the early high priests of medicine, a modern *curandero*.)

37. In the early rush for patients, some programs grew large, while others broke into one or two new mutualities. This process was favored by the medical strikes, which divided the staff of each service into different groups. When strikers formed new clinics, their orientation was directed toward their previous patients. The economic depression of the thirties reduced the number of paying patients (who reverted to the public system, always a backup for mutualism) while it encouraged the work of new mutualities. To offer but one example, the Centro Balear, with 12,000 members in 1932, ended its existence in February 1933 after seven months of strikes. Its staff subdivided and formed four new clinics: (1) Asociación Clínica de La Habana, by the home physicians; (2) Asociación Nuestra Señora del Pilar, by the clinical and hospital staff; (3) Centro Nuevo, by the physicians of the executive committee; and (4) Asociación La Bien Aparecida, by the members of the executive committee who withdrew before the strike. See Leland, p. 94.

38. Dechamp and Troncoso, p. 17.

39. Taking advantage of ethnic conflict, some clinics, like the Policlínica Nacional Cubana and its "surgeon-director" (and enemy of Acción Inmediata) Nicolás Gómez de Rosas sought to attract patients who were uncomfortable with the Spanish identity of larger programs.

40. The Casino Español of the Centro Asturiano has been qualified, for example, as the "heart of reaction and conservatism." See Commission on Cuban Affairs, *Problems of the New Cuba* (Wilson George Smillie, primary author of section on public health), (New York: Foreign Policy Association, 1935), p. 39.

41. A term which appears (in translation) in a speech of Fidel Castro on the occasion of the opening of the polyclinic in the community of Valle del Perú, *Granma* (January 19, 1969): 2.

42. Relations between private, mutualist, and public hospitals were chaotic in any case, with whole blocks of subscribers bought and sold among different plans. The public service was not so much an alternative source of care; it was a public subsidy for private practice and mutualism, which sent all uncomfortable cases to public facilities or used public facilities for the work of the mutualities.

43. Interview with a physician, highly placed in the prerevolutionary university.

44. Still, the official figures of 1934 may hide certain hidden employment by "voluntary" physicians or represent a recent improvement. Leland, p. 94, found physicians in 1933 on the staff of large clinics at $25 per month while a very few earned $350 per month.

45. This, incidentally, became the long range objective, recently achieved, of the revolutionary government after 1959.

46. Fernández-Conde, p. 59. Aldereguía later became a distinguished physician and has served as ambassador to Yugoslavia under the socialist government.

47. Ibid., p. 56.

48. "Immobility" does not really mean immobility; rather it prescribed a "due process" that effectively gave final authority to the FMC in matters of employer-employee conflict.

49. Thomas, p. 765.

50. José Antonio Presno Bastiony had the good fortune to marry the daughter of Cuba's most eminent surgeon, the great urologist Joaquín Albarrán, professor in Paris at the turn of the twentieth century. See J. Paulís Pagés and M.Y. Monteros-Valdivieso, *Joaquín Albarrán: general artífice de la urología* (Havana: Museo Histórico de las Ciencias Médicas "Carlos J. Finlay," 1963), p. 75.

51. A gynecologist who brought together the two most eminent medical names in Pinar del Río, Gustavo Cuervo Rubio headed for many years the department of gynecology in Mercedes hospital and held a professorship in the university. See also Thomas, pp. 656, 678, and 982.

52. See Thomas, pp. 740-43 and 764.

53. For a general discussion of the prerevolutionary structure of government-supported health services, complete with organizational charts, see: Cuba. Ministerio de Salud Pública, Subsecretaria de Economía, *Publicación No. 1, Datos y cifras en salud pública, 1962* (pamphlet), (Havana: Ministerio de Salud Pública, n.d.), pp. 1-4. It mentions one additional category of services that is not mentioned here, the private infirmaries of the largest sugar mills.

54. The Colegio Médico de La Habana listed five Antonettis in 1945: Juan A. Antonetti Fernández, Melba Antonetti Fernández, Alfredo Antonetti Muñiz, Carlos C. Antonetti Muñiz, and Alfredo Antonetti Vivar. The elder Alfredo Antonetti emigrated in 1968 after the budget of mutualism was incorporated in the Ministry of Public Health in 1967. See *Relación de Médicos, 1945*.

55. A rare copy of a recent historical study of the Centro Benéfico de los Trabajadores de Cuba remains confiscated by U.S. Customs. Other reference may be found in Gómez Luaces, pp. 38-39.

56. Data derived from a study of family budgets conducted by the Banco Nacional de Cuba in 1952, cited by Jacinto Torras, "Los factores económicos en la crisis médica," *Economía y Desarrollo* 3 (July-August 1973) 4: 21.

6
Early Transition Under the Socialist Revolution

The dusty and difficult trek of the poor from Havana to Mercedes Hospital had been transformed, in the course of seventy years, into a popular casino and hotel-lined thoroughfare to the heart of fashionable Vedado. The immediate vicinity of the hospital had become a favored location for the city's prestigious medical offices. By taking advantage of skyrocketing real estate values in the 1950s, Mercedes Hospital was able to sell its site in Vedado and construct a new facility on land provided by the city. But the events of 1959 thwarted the plans to erect high-rise commercial buildings on the old site. The unoccupied land was soon destined as the site of the revolution's ice cream parlor, Copelia. More than fifty flavors may now be consumed in the healthy location recommended by Tomás Romay for the quarantine of new immigrants.

Diagonally across from the remains of Las Mercedes, the towering Hilton Hotel saw its name changed to Libre, while two blocks down the thoroughfare, the reorganized Ministry of Health and Social Assistance moved into an office building belonging to the Cuban Medical Federation. At the same time, logically, revolutionaries and progressives began to move from the federation to the ministry. This process brought new conflicts to the federation. In 1960, Acción Inmediata fell under the influence of physicians who opposed government actions which they believed compromised the autonomy of the profession. Supporters of the government responded by forming still another medical party, the Party of the Revolution. Gathering their forces, the Revolution Party won control of the federation in 1961. Not long thereafter, in 1963, the federation declared itself made obsolete by the revolution and ended its existence formally in 1966. The principal functions of the federation were replaced by a medical workers' union and scientific associations. The decision to disband the federation was an expression of the impatience with which the revolutionary leadership viewed the old conflicts of the profession. Furthermore, the events of the first three years, including the emigration of one-third of Cuba's physicians by the end of 1963, did render the federation obsolete. To appreciate how this was the case, and also to appreciate the disgruntlement of unhappy physicians, it is necessary to examine the early revolution and its implications for the prerevolutionary medical class.

THE CUBAN REVOLUTION

The Rebel Army marched into Havana in January 1959 with a substantial component of medical workers, physicians, and students. They were cheered by the throngs which filled the streets and also by the Cuban Medical Federation. The revolutionaries, in their turn, saluted the medical profession: "Of all the professions," Ché Guevara remarked before an assembly of the federation, "It is the medical profession which has given most to the Revolution."[1] Indeed, in the previous years, the federation had openly opposed the Batista dictatorship. Under the leadership of Acción Inmediata, the federation enjoined the International Red Cross to investigate Batista's repression of physicians who dared give medical assistance to wounded insurgents. The investigation discredited the Batista regime and facilitated the supply of medical aid to the rebels.

Insurgent participation by the medical profession was perfectly consistent with the class character of the early rebellion, which united all progressives against the tyranny. Once again in 1957-58, as in the prelude to the fall of Machado, the university was closed while many students and faculty joined the opposition. The Cuban Revolution emerged from a rural constituency and took hold in an ideologically developed working class, but it was also substantially supported by the progressives within the professional and privileged classes.[2] Unlike the experience of the 1930s, this time the revolution would sustain a consistent direction for the creative energy awakened in the rebellion. But while the revolution gave structure to professional idealism, the speed of events and escalating socialist ideology, combined with the profound ambiguities within the medical profession, determined that the revolution would contain two processes of conflict within the medical sector—the polarization within the medical "class" and the transformation of the class content of medical work. Notwithstanding the harmony of interests expressed in the encounter between Guevara and the federation, the medical profession had at least as many differences in 1959 as it had in 1933. And to these differences were added others: Batista collaborators versus noncollaborators, revolutionaries versus nonrevolutionaries, and revolutionaries versus counterrevolutionaries. These terms, coined in the heat of conflict and movement, swept aside more precise categories. Physicians who were hurt or confused by the speed of events, which made life difficult for everyone, had little time to comprehend the revolution or find their own compromise before they were recruited *en masse* to the United States.

While some physicians immediately fled the country, others—activists in the urban underground, revolutionary sympathizers, and, of course, ordinary opportunists—were busily donning rebel army fatigues. An activist from the urban underground, Saturnino Paez, was named to head the Ministry of Health and Social Assistance, and he proceeded to brusquely purge Batista's appointees. Rebel physicians were named to sanitary posts and to hospital directorships; while the new Mercedes Hospital was renamed to honor the martyred rebel army physician, Manuel Fajardo.

In the beginning the revolution was not socialist, communist, or self-consciously social democratic. The social reformism, such as that expressed in Fidel Castro's famous defense after the 1953 attack on the Moncada barracks in Santiago, was uncompromisingly oriented to seeking solutions to the social, economic, and health problems of rural and poor Cuba. An important context for such reform was determined by a history of political struggles of an urban proletariat and a very large rural proletariat that had been led for years by Marxist unions. The new revolutionary government immediately instituted liberal social reforms, such as the agrarian reforms which broadened land ownership, and the urban reforms which halved or abolished rents on most housing. These measures, and the literacy campaign of 1961, produced early success and a great deal of popular enthusiasm. But as development progressed—as quick pay-off measures and short-run planning gave way to long-run strategies, as problematic outcomes of early solutions thrust themselves increasingly on the political agenda, and as the United States intensified its hostility toward Cuba—traditional reforms seemed insufficient to the revolutionary leaders. Finally, Cuba embraced socialism, with unintended help by the United States and with very intentional assistance from the world socialist community. Key ingredients of the revolution seem to me to have been, from the beginning, the following: (1) commitment to very basic social change, favoring the rural and poorer classes, (2) pragmatic assessment of the role of the United States, (3) determination to develop the Rebel Army and the militia, and (4) recognition of the role of the Cuban Communist party and its allies.

The problems of the health system that the revolution inherited were essentially the features that already predominated in the 1930s and were clearly enunciated in the 1934 report of the International Labor Office[3] and other early studies. Their concerns were echoed in 1957, when the Cuban Medical Federation celebrated a national conference on the "medical crisis."[4] One resolution proposed that new mutualist clinics should not be permitted in towns of Cuba which already had such plans; another resolution favored more vigorous government action against unauthorized practitioners. Both the conference of 1957 and the report of 1934 made ample use of the expression "plethora of physicians in Havana," a set of words which at once suggests the underlying urban-rural contradiction, and the antagonism within the medical profession between a privileged minority and the marginal majority. Considering the wealth of prerevolutionary analysis, it is interesting to note the degree to which the first directions and values of health promotion under the revolution have their origins, first, in the frustrated prerevolutionary consciousness of health advocates and, second, in the conflicts and antagonisms that are intensified within the process of the revolution. Once discovers that, as early changes produced their own contradictions within the revolution, new directions were increasingly signaled by concepts and norms that do not antedate the revolution itself.

In the following pages, I will sketch the outlines that I have uncovered of early development under the revolution, organizing my discussion by institutional subdivisions of the health sector. Early transformations include the period from 1959 to 1964. I interpret the years 1965 through 1971 as a period of consolidation. And the years after 1971 have reason to be called the period of medicine in the community.

The most important health effort of the new government in 1959 was clearly the building of a rural health service. This was followed in 1961 by the expulsion of old leadership from the medical school and in 1962 by the reorganization of the ministry of health. Nonetheless, it must be understood that while the rural service and other new Cuban departures were being established, the institutions of mutualism, the mainstream of previous health care development in Cuba, were omnipresent as ever in Havana and growing in the early revolutionary environment. In a sense, the predominant developments in health services *encircled* mutualism, with the revolution striking more directly at rural Cuba, major public institutions, and the medical school. Therefore, the account of changes in mutualism will follow an account of changes external to mutualism that were the central developments of the new Cuban health system. By trying to keep in mind an uninterrupted role of mutualism, one is more likely to avoid the extreme emphasis on the break with the past.

RURAL HEALTH SERVICE

At the turn of the present century, when rural Cuba lay devastated by years of cruel warfare with Spain, the meaning of the urban-rural dichotomy was suddenly and profoundly altered by metropolitan sanitary improvements and the end of the great urban epidemics.[5] In earlier times, it was commonplace for the rich to flee Havana for the more healthy environment of rural Cuba. But a new perspective on rural Cuba was probably retarded by the impression that rural problems were a passing circumstance of war, and the reality of rural life was hidden, throughout the presocialist period, by the inadequacy of rural morbidity statistics, itself a consequence of nonexistent services. While the reach of a considerable and well-intentioned sanitary movement among physicians was restrained by ineffective and disinterested government, the majority of physicians were blinded to rural needs by a predominantly curative[6] and individualistic, not to say capitalistic,[7] medical orientation as well as by their own urban middle class origins.

As with sanitary services, the always increasing value of clinical medicine was withheld from the rural population for two principle reasons: the variable poverty of rural Cuba generated insufficient and irregular real demand for the physician's services, and the small rural towns seldom offered conditions for middle class life that were regarded as essential for a physician and his family. Yet, it was precisely in the many small towns where the services of physician and sanitarian were most urgently needed.[8] Unable to effect changes in these conditions, and without the means to transcend such difficulties, it was without effect that the report of the International Labor Office clearly stated in 1933 that one way to resolve the "plethora" of physicians in Havana was to move them to the interior. In 1935, the Commission on Cuban Affairs of the Foreign Policy Association stated the problem most succinctly:

> Cuba is training more physicians than the island can possibly utilize *under the present plan of private practice of medicine* and the probable course of economic development of the country.
>
> But there exists relative scarcity of physicians in the interior where the need is greatest, and a great overabundance of physicians in the capital. With each annual increase of young medical graduates, conditions will continue to grow worse.
>
> The difficulty is that no system has been devised whereby the great mass of Cuban people who live in the interior and really need good medical and hospital service can secure it.[9]

While these words lost some of their force as Cuba slowly climbed out of the depression years, they lost none of their validity. They were underscored in 1953 by the national census and again in 1957 by a survey of rural Cuba that was conducted by the Agrupación Católica Universitaria.[10]

While the emphasis on rural development by the new government constituted a rather complete break with the past, it is more accurate to say that what was previously a minority concern became a majoritarian effort. Indeed, the "rural problem" had been a constant Cuban preoccupation not unlike or unrelated to an earlier preoccupation with slavery. Among the medical ranks, a special concern for rural health had been maintained by an important nucleus of physicians who developed the specialty of tropical medicine and parasitology, as the two were customarily combined. Many health problems treated under this heading were most critical among the rural population and urban poor. Here the advances of treatment methodologies were frustrated by the nonpaying characteristic of patients and by the greater probability of reinfestation or reinfection. The nature of the field, therefore, caused its students to be sensitive to the need for an integration of sanitary and preventive measures with inexpensive or free curative services. Their medical ideology became, so to speak, that of "social medicine". The pages of the *Revista KUBA de Medicina Tropical y de Parisitología* chronicled, after 1944, the distribution of parasites and other diseases among the rural population. By 1959, there was no extreme shortage of medical understanding of rural pathologies.

Early Plans for Rural Health Centers

The importance of previous development of tropical and social medicine in giving orientation to the new Cuban health system is suggested by the many features of the contemporary Cuban "model" that appeared in the very first plans for the rural health service. An example is the plan authored by Rafael Calvó Fonseca[11] and the Finlay Institute[12] that was published in *Revista KUBA* in early 1959. The plan apparently had a semiofficial character, carrying as it did the name of a research arm of the ministry of health. Central to the plan was the concept of a rural health center which would integrate prevention and cure, medicine and sanitation, physician and health team, and professional and lay participation in health work. The centers would replace or supplement the long degraded system of municipal sanitary chiefs. They would establish, in the military terms that have since lent an epic spirit to the Cuban battle against disease, beachheads of modern services in the rural environment. Thus, in unmistakable terms, the plan of rural services emphasized the *periphery* of services: "Here we are working in reverse; instead of carrying health from the center to the periphery, we intend to begin with the periphery, establishing these modern services of health."[13]

Minimally, the center would employ a physician who would serve as director, a visiting nurse, a midwife, and a laboratory technician who would also serve as sanitary inspector. The first task of the new physician was to carry out a sociomedical survey of the area. Officials, teachers, and important farmers were to be visited and a census made of midwives and folk healers. Previously existing data on births, deaths, and morbidity were to be gathered from every possible source, and, the proposal suggested, a large map of the area could be constructed and posted in a prominent wall of the new facility. Armed with such a beginning, the next step for the new physician-director was to initiate a program of meetings with specific groups, such as the Parents and Teachers Association, making sure that other revolutionary officials of the area also attend the meetings in order to convincingly indicate the social importance of the new center and of the meetings themselves. Thus, an idea emerged that would later yield results beyond any original expectation. The purpose of social relations between health center and community was not simply to gain passive acceptance or to alter beliefs; the larger aim was to *organize the community for active participation in health promotion:*

> It will turn out convenient, after a certain time has passed and the neighbors of the zone are impressed by the work carried out, to build Health Councils . . . or whatever they may be called, formed by representative persons of the zone (and with these Committees we have magnificent personal experience), thus obtaining citizen cooperation and erasing the incomprehension and indifference— when not the hostility—with which such efforts are received in many places where illiteracy and absurd beliefs stand in the way of sanitary measures. This social action would help neighbors cooperate in the protection and development of their own health and that of the community.[14]

If one may judge from reports published by the first rural physicians, it seems that the elements of the plan presented above correspond closely to the practice that developed.[15]

First Experience of the Rural Health Service

The rapid construction of rural facilities indicated the strength of government commitment and its impact on physicians who were drawn to rural service. By 1963, 122 rural centers and 42 rural hospitals with a combined total of 1,155 beds were established, employing in 1963 some 322 physicians and 49 dentists.[16] Taking into account some variation in the time spent per physician in rural service, the number of physicians who, by 1963, had performed rural service was much larger than the 322 positions budgeted in 1963. Law 723 of 1960 obligated medical graduates to spend one year in rural service, and, by 1963, 1,500 physicians and 50 dentists were estimated to have experienced rural service.[17] Besides the direct impact of the rural program on physicians; hospitals, medical associations, and the medical school were asked to develop programs which would support the rural effort.

On the one hand, the rural service effectively constituted a national experiment in tropical and social medicine. On the other hand—since the context was a snowballing program of agrarian reform, mass mobilization, and the preoccupations of a popular movement threatened from abroad— many physicians effectively became medical *cadre*, in the sense that their work became a part of a politically defined organization, life style, and personal identity. The revolutionary integration of the health enterprise was not a mere formality. After all, many of the rural facilities were actually built by the National Institute for Agrarian Reform (INRA), the politically conscious umbrella organization that implemented the program of agrarian reform. Often, the supplies of rural facilities came from INRA, and where there were no pharmacies, or inadequate pharmacies, the new people's stores served this purpose. When the health center sought community cooperation, the center was logically directed toward the organizations created by the revolution which were effecting such participation. Thus, the stint of the rural physician could not help but be, in addition to a course in tropical and social medicine, a course in political economy and social dynamics.[18]

A turning point—when this revolutionary, tropical, or social medicine became *Cuban* medicine, or at least a self-conscious vanguard of Cuban medicine—was the Tenth National Medical Congress held in Havana, February 17-24, 1963, and attended by some 2,000 physicians. Prominent among the approximately 600 papers presented at the congress were reports by physicians of the rural health service. Here the rural pathologies, whose broad features had been sketched before 1959 but had to be rediscovered, with difficulty, by each medical generation, now appeared in the intimate terms of the community case study and direct experience serving rural health needs. One report offered a conclusion that has become a basic tenet of contemporary health practice: "The local mass organizations are our best aid in the arduous task of elevating the sanitary level of the zone . . . The physician, faced by the magnitude of these tasks, can only be coordinator, orientor of this mass."[19] A newly-bearded physician, thus situated, could not fail to see his own efforts as only one part of a set of health-related measures: land reform, new roads, improved agricultural methods, schools, literacy programs, improved diet, and an end to seasonal unemployment—"sacred obligations contracted by the troops of the Liberation Army."[20]

MEDICAL SCHOOL

The University of Havana was, in 1959, the most influential institution of the Cuban professional class: alma mater to most, an employer and instrument of its elite, and a mold for future members. The most influential physicians seldom failed to have faculty appointments (some of them for generations) and physicians with faculty appointments seldom failed to be influential or prosperous in their profession. The rocky transition of the university is of special interest, then, because it reveals contradictory meanings that the revolution spelled for Cuban professionals. Medical education was profoundly changed in the first years of the Cuban Revolution. Its principal features by 1963 reflected the new general features of the university:

1. a change in the social origin of students, inspired by free tuition, residential scholarships, and political incentives;
2. the implementation of the contract system in faculty employment, thus terminating the much abused and unwieldy system of *concurso-oposición* and fifth year "evaluation";
3. student and national government authority in university administration, thus ending the formal hegemony of the faculty in university affairs and also the formal autonomy of the university;
4. a great expansion of the university budget, designed to favor practical human resource needs of the society;
5. the frequent employment of foreign and young Cuban professors to replace the large number of prerevolutionary professors who ended their work during the first years of educational reorganization; and
6. the constant visible presence of the revolution in the university, manifested in new organizations, the student and faculty militia, the new Federation of University Students, and others.

Specifically, medical education changed in the following ways:

1. an increase in the number of teaching hospitals from four to seven, and the establishment of a medical school in the Universities of Las Villas and Santiago de Cuba;
2. the incorporation of hospital internship as a prerequisite for graduation;
3. the creation of a new school of preclinical sciences for the first two years of medical education;
4. an early curriculum emphasis, consistent with compulsory rural service, on epidemiology, statistics, social medicine, including health services administration, and rural or tropical medicine; and
5. a crash program to greatly increase the number of Cuban physicians.

To an outside observer, the changes that were effected by 1963, in curriculum, departmental organization, and student careers, may not seem extreme. But the rapid and impatient changes overstepped cumbersome procedural regulations and thus raised conflicts with professional associations and their privileged immobility, while government involvement violated the grand ideal of university autonomy. That is, the revolution assaulted the very ideals that were considered in the prerevolutionary period victories of the Cuban professional and medical class.

Antagonism between the Revolution and the Old University

The new goals of the health sector, the rural service in particular, pressured changes in medical training. The number of rural physicians could hardly be increased by graduating medical students who were, almost without exception, from the urban middle class. New physicians could hardly be expected to perform in the isolated conditions of rural service if their training remained highly verbalistic and theoretical, sometimes without clinical contacts until the fourth year. And few students could emerge as effective general physicians if their clinical training in the last years of medical school was heavily concentrated in a single specialty, under the tutelage of a single professor. If there were so few internships (less than 30 for an average class of nearly 200), students would continue to be ill-prepared for modern hospital work that rested on collaboration among various health workers, specialists and professions. New physicians would fail to acquire the diagnostic familiarity that was essential in rural service. Important branches of medical science such as biochemistry, totally absent in the prerevolutionary school, needed to be added to the curriculum, but in which of the jealous departments should they be included, if new departments and institutes were opposed?

The problem faced by reform in medical education is suggested by the despair with which the previous social democratic governments of Grau San Martín and Prío Socarrás had regarded medical education. As a highly positioned official of those years, now in the U.S., remarked, the only feasible way within the old system to change education was to build an entirely new school.[21]

University and professional autonomy, before 1959, had served different interests, uniting all who feared the vicissitudes of government and valued the role of the university as a somewhat detached critic of government and society. But it is also true to say that, by 1959, the concept of autonomy had lost much of its intrinsic appeal through years of abuse by Cuban government and by the professors and professionals themselves. The always insufficient financial support and indirect intervention by government reinforced the islands of authoritarian self-sufficiency of some faculty, and the network of favoritism that linked them to a mass of part-time appointments. In the lumbering giant that the university had become, autonomy no longer suggested the positive or dynamic quality it may once have promised; autonomy was correctly confused with the negative concept of immobility. Moreover, the great popularity of the revolution undermined the fundamental preconditions for such ideals: fear of government, perceived discontinuity between government and public interests, the social alienation of intellectuals. Thus, by mid-1960 active support for the old system was bound to be concentrated in an easily isolated group: independently powerful faculty, strict proceduralists, and anticommunists. In large measure, the old ideals simply disappeared, and a new concept of the university integrated into the revolution emerged, with new ideals.

The threatened end of autonomy and of *concurso-oposición* (the much abused method of verbal contests for vacant faculty positions) and other proposals of university reform divided the medical faculty and the active members of the Cuban Medical Federation, some of whom were already taken aback by the purge of the prestigious administrative committees in Calixto García and other public hospitals. Thus, when the medical faculty was convened on the evening of July 29, 1960, to decide its posture vis á vis a newly formed revolutionary Superior Governing Board for the university, the faculty was evenly divided on the issue.[22] A few days later, the Superior Governing Board was provisionally recognized by the revolutionary government. Some professors were fired, others left the university in protest, and new professors were appointed. Finally, in laws enacted in 1961, numerous structural reforms and the direct participation in university affairs by the Ministry of Education, alongside evenly weighted student and faculty representation, was instituted.[23]

Actually, what existed were two rather different processes, both racing against the other and destined to conflict: the process of reconsolidating the old university after its two years of interruption, and the process of the revolution itself. Because the latter was barely beginning in early 1959, the first confrontation could only seek to eliminate the more obvious elements that had been tarnished by Batista and to propose changes that were reasonable by consensual prerevolutionary standards. This process was speedily carried out in the spirit of returning to work and led to an agreement on new statutes that was approved, it seems, by the Student Federation, leading the established faculty to reasonably anticipate their much desired return to normalcy. However, by July 1960, a genuine revolution was intensifying, acquiring greater solidarity, organization, and direction. Attention could thus shift, at some point, from *batistianos* to counterrevolutionaries and from "what is needed to make the university function" to "what is needed to make the revolution."

The indignant response by some Cuban faculty cannot surprise anyone who has witnessed the anxieties of faculties disrupted by student protests of the last decade in the United States. Where these and other efforts have been directed toward university reforms—open admission, special programs for disadvantaged students, curricular innovation, changes in grading methods, departmental reorganization, student and junior faculty power in governance, the increased employment of women and third world minorities—senior faculty members have everywhere formed the strongest opposition.[24]

Emergence of the New University

The situation was not so different in Cuba. Large numbers of scholarship students entered the university, most of them not from Havana. The number of poor, rural, nonwhite and women students greatly increased. For many reasons, including the fact that the best preuniversity high schools were in Havana, the new students were less prepared academically than the traditional middle class students of Havana, thus raising the spectre among faculty and middle class students of declining quality of education and lowered standards. The new students were, however, ideologically superior and conscious of their role as the youth of the revolution. To some, the new students were feared as "red thugs."[25] Without doubt, many of the new students, and not a few "old" students, must have soon become as vigilant in detecting reactionary and counter-revolutionary ideas as militant black students are sometimes vigilant in detecting racist ideas and practices in many Northern American universities, much to the distress of many professors and fellow students. As one middle class former medical student, now in the United States, put it, "We knew who each other were, and they were always suspicious of us."

From these comments that suggest a clear class conflict within the university, one may correctly anticipate that on one level the conflict between university professionals and the revolution took the form of a *cultural* conflict. The nostalgic decorum of a "bicentennial" university was shattered by the new revolutionaries.[26] Thus, in reference to the armed occupation of the university by students in January and February of 1959, a senior member of the medical faculty wrote, with the characteristic note of injured dignity and pride:

> Professorial authority was left seriously stained and many professors who for their experience and executive ability should have been the directors of University Reform were left on the side, separated by an abyss of unresolvable incomprehension, on being confronted by a student mob, whose passions had been demogogically exalted.[27]

The University Council was appalled as much by the disrespectful tone of student manifestos as by the demands presented therein. Indeed, a way of life was threatened, it seemed, and "culture was offended." Of the new university, the same professor added:

even the gallant and suggestive whistle has been quieted. How could one whistle at the [woman] militia comrade who boasts of hate, of absence of every feminine sentiment and, on top of all this, of filth, with her pride diverted by consuming no more than one bar of soap per month, by not using deodorant, perfume, or other articles which, disrespectfully called bourgeois, contribute so much to achieve the enchantment of femininity.[28]

Such pedestrian concerns suggest that the departure of faculty and middle class students or, more correctly in my view, the rout of Cuban physicians into emigration, is not to be explained simply by reference to new policies of curriculum, organization, and governance. (After all, there was no great emigration of faculty when the university was closed by Batista.) Rather, the rout of Cuban physicians, like the rout of the middle class as a whole, is explained by the escalating social turmoil and speed of the larger revolution. In a country whose fate had turned for the previous one hundred years on the approval and disapproval of the United States, only the most imaginative of the older middle class could suppose that hostility with the United States would not end in the demise of the revolution.

My conclusion is that many emigrés were less reactionary than naively opportunistic and, had they had more time and been less pressured by the escalation of events, could have found a useful niche, and reconciliation with the revolution.

While the period of turbulent polarization peaked in 1961 with the defeated Bay of Pigs invasion and continued through the great missile crisis of October 1962, physicians who stayed or who joined the faculty of the university in this period found a remarkably different university. The departure of professors and many middle class students created an impact well beyond the effects of their numbers.[29] Perhaps two-thirds of the old medical faculty and one-third of Cuba's physicians had left the country by 1963. But the loss of faculty had one profound effect—aside, one might be tempted to quip, from reducing the "plethora" of physicians. It created a profound sense of solidarity amidst an embattled university within an embattled and righteous society. In this solidarity, the exaggerated social distance between students and faculty was reduced out of necessity. From the milieu of new social contacts—militia, voluntary labor, membership on committees and political groups—came endless meetings. The sense of equality of comrades-in-arms was imperceptibly merged in the title of *compañero* with the ideology of equality among men and women under socialism. As the university adopted an identity as a socialist university (another term in an already rich vocabulary of revolution) the departure of physicians left an unmistakable image of the prerevolutionary physician that would be recalled to future generations of medical students. *His private self interest was placed above the exercise of his art; he abandoned his country in its hour of need.*

Thus, the flight of physicians, and great polarization, gave substance to a developing counterconcept of the new physician: Unlike the old physician, the new physician would be formed according to the needs of the society, interpreted by the revolution, and would practice where the need, not the profit, was the greatest. Or as many students were by then saying, "wherever the revolution sends me." Considering that emigré physicians included prominent figures in private practice who seemed to have left their country in pursuit of economic gain, it was not inconsistent that the new physician also renounced private practice, suddenly the symbol of medicine "before the revolution."

The changing social origins of students, already noted, was greatly intensified, first, as a direct consequence of the departure of many middle class students, and second, as a consequence of the dramatic response of the revolutionary government to the departure of physicians. In a celebrated speech of 1962, Fidel Castro analyzed the "shameful" flight of physicians and called on revolutionary youth, workers and students, to volunteer for medical training. The call found an enthusiastic response in the university, in the high schools, and among working youth. Students in law, humanities, and social studies transferred to medicine, while many high school students decided on a medical career. But almost half of the students in the first year class in autumn 1963 were working youths, many of whom were given special preuniversity courses before entering the medical program proper.[30]

New students then, in 1963, had not simply chosen a medical career; they had been called by the revolution. The new class of over 1,000 students consciously perceived itself as different from earlier students, and was born amid the pains of a new society with a sense of mission that derived directly from the antagonisms within the old medical class. The new students of 1963 were destined to celebrate the tenth anniversary of the Triumph of the Rebellion with their entrance to internship programs. In the ensuing years, their presence in the university would set the tone of student life and medical education. After 1962, the medical program itself would be consciously preparing students for a new political and social role. This meant that seminars on Marxist social analysis and guerilla warfare would be part of premedical training, lectures might lapse into political discussions, and technical visits to new facilities would always include a nontechnical reminder of how things were before the revolution. Someday, the 1963 Cuban report to the World Health Organization announced, Cuba would offer medical assistance to other countries "in process of liberation."[31]

University training and medical work was internationalized in the course of these transformations. Foreign medical workers from twenty-six nations were contracted by the Ministry of Public Health, 120 in 1964 and 92 in 1965. Most came from Argentina, Mexico, and Ecuador, followed by Bulgaria, the Soviet Union, Czechoslavakia, and Hungary. Meanwhile, 118 scholarship students were abroad for specialty training in the 1964-1965 academic year, most of them to socialist countries. In 1964-1965, Cubans participated in fifty-six conferences in thirty-one nations.[32] And an interesting political advertisement appeared in the *Tribuna Médica* in 1963: a proclamation of solidarity with the MPLA, the Popular Movement for the Liberation of Angola.

While there were no women on the medical faculty in 1958, there were a dozen in 1963. In all its history, the University of Havana graduated 696 female physicians, 200 of them in the years 1959 through 1963.[33]

Other responses by the university to the flight of physicians included a reduction of the preinternship period from six to four years and from four to three years in dentistry. Where emigration seriously affected specialties, medical students were recruited to vertical internships that offered early specialty certification. These changes were reversed in 1965, the year which definitively ends the first period of transition. Preinternship curriculum was extended to five years, and the escalated verticle internship was abandoned in favor of the rotating internship for generalists that was already compulsory for other students. The improved internship and clinical years were made possible by the greatly expanded organization of teaching functions in Havana hospitals, and by the sharpened definition of preclinical studies in the new preclinical center. It is also true to say that the first few years, through 1963, were marked by a somewhat cavalier disregard, probably impossible to avoid in the circumstances that have been described, of certain scientific concerns, methodology of scientific research, and research itself.[34] With the exception of increased attention to the various topics of social medicine, the curriculum itself was not greatly changed, and the work of different departments, on the concrete level, continued to be performed in relative isolation. This characteristic, not uncommon to other medical schools, probably continued to be influenced by the organization and facilities of the principal university hospital, Calixto Garcia, which was actually a cluster of separate little hospitals. Moreover, the improvisation required to keep each department functioning and staffed with competent personnel gave little opportunity to develop a perspective, much less a really new perspective, of the whole enterprise of medical education.

Tropical and Social Medicine

An exception was found in the teaching of parasitology and tropical and social medicine, where solid roots for new reforms were found in a prerevolutionary minority critique of medical education. In 1952 the teaching of social medicine had been found "denaturalized" by "professionalism" and reduced to "so many prescriptions of sanitation." The curriculum should seek instead, the critics argued,

> the spiritual preparation to comprehend the elevated mission that belongs to social and preventive medicine . . . and to develop an essentially statistical vision of life in all its manifestation.[35]

Before 1959, a short course on social medicine was offered in the last year of the medical curriculum, after the clinical formation of the student was complete. After 1959, this course was superseded by a program for each year, beginning with statistical methodology, passing through biostatistics and epidemiology, and ending in the last year with health care organization. The courses included field trips and, in the first year, a course in family health, where students personally investigated the living conditions of patients discharged from university hospitals.[36] Meanwhile the spiritual formation for social medicine merged with ideological formation, or, alternatively, social medicine acquired the characteristic of official ideology.

Clearly related to social medicine, the Cuban specialty of tropical medicine was greatly developed after 1940 under the aegis of the Instituto de Parisitología y de Medicina Tropical.[37] But while Cuban tropical medicine and parasitology gained scientific respect in Cuba and among Latin American colleagues, its actual influence was small on the overall orientation of medicine and medical training. Medical students everywhere, after all, create order out of the mammoth enterprise of medical education by focusing on those aspects which seem most relevant to career anticipations. Yet, it was precisely the career anticipations that were soon to change dramatically in Cuba: first to rural service, compulsory for graduates after 1960; second, away from private practice to salaried work within an organized setting, compulsory for students graduating after 1965; and third, to the provision of primary levels of health care rather than exclusive specialization. Logically, the expansion of the curriculum in tropical medicine was one of the first new characteristics of the reopened university in 1959.

EMERGING NATIONAL HEALTH SYSTEM

In 1959, when the Ministry of Public Health was given broad powers in matters related to health services, few could have anticipated how far this authority would be used to create a new health system. Excepting the new services to rural Cuba, no new organizational direction was apparent for health services as a system. Quite in line with normal expectations, the power of the Ministry was first used to purge *batistianos* and sinecures, while the administration of some important hospitals, and the ministry itself, was turned over to physicians who had served in the rebel army and to other trusted physicians. In the meantime, the social bias, if not the precise direction, of changes to come was suggested in legislation to lower the price of medicines and medical accessories[38] and of course by the rural program, whose broad implications were not immediately visible.

In 1961, at a turning point in Cuban history, the first plan began to take form for a comprehensive national system of health services. This plan, implemented in 1962 and significantly revised in 1965, included many of the formal structural features that are part of the present Cuban system. It created decentralized provincial and regional levels, responsible for concrete administration and planning, and a national level responsible for norms and orientation. All levels integrated the functions of public health: treatment, health protection, long and short range planning, and scientific improvement of health workers. The new structure of public health activities is summarized in Diagram 6.1.

Diagram 6.1
Principal Organizational Categories of
MINSAP, 1962

Hierarchy-Levels of Organization and Administration

	Responsible for Norms and Orientation	Responsible for Concrete Administration and Planning	
	NATIONAL	PROVINCIAL (7-also called regions)	REGIONAL (126-also called zones)
CURATIVE FUNCTIONS	Subministry of Medical Assistance	Same Subsection; Administer Provincial Hospital; Oversee all services	Same Subsection; Administer Regional Hospitals; Oversee all services
HEALTH PROTECTION	Subministry of Hygiene and Epidemiology	Centers of Hygiene and Epidemiology	Centers (same)
LONG AND SHORT RANGE PLANNING, BUDGETING	Subministry of Economics and Planning	Same Subsection	Same Subsection
SCIENTIFIC IMPROVEMENT OF HEALTH WORKERS	Scientific Council, societies, committees, task forces	Committees, Task Forces	Committees, Task Forces

Integrated Functions of Public Health

Although the first plan appears to be a close adaptation of the Czech variant of East European and Soviet models,[39] it is clear that some form of national health planning was in any case called for by Cuban experience from 1959 to 1961. The increased mobilization and military organization of Cuban society, the socialist declaration, the open role of aid from socialist countries, and the high tide of internal political polarization all favored the introduction of the most comprehensively nationalized system at a time when the health system itself was already leaning in this direction. Assuming continuity of power by the revolutionary government, the initial phase of quantitative efforts was bound to pressure also the qualitative change involving organization and planning on the level of the whole system.

It is easy to see how the new structure of administration sometimes has had the appearance of an arbitrary expression of new Soviet influence and socialist formulas. Like many incorrect impressions, there was some truth involved. The new socialist period from 1961 to 1963, increased the influence of many who sometimes applied the Czech model in a rather mechanical fashion. Detailed progress reports were frequently required of the new provincial and regional administrations, including categories of information that were of no operational interest to the national office and sometimes beyond the capacity of lower units to provide.[40] Although the model prescribed a rule of "normative centralization and administrative decentralization," it was hardly clear what this meant for the precise relation between the national and provincial offices in a very new system. Should the Cubans begin where the developed Czech system had already arrived? Were the new norms of health work sufficiently understood so that one could have confidence in real decentralization? Perhaps new procedures seemed arbitrary and bureaucratic because few understood them. Not unexpectedly, the commitment by national administration to organization, procedure, and rational, systematic planning as the sine qua non of modern and socialist health promotion created conflict between those whose immediate concern was the construction of a new system and those whose immediate concern was the direct delivery of services and administration of specific facilities.

Prerevolutionary and New Revolutionary Antagonisms

This conflict between unit and system was resolved by 1965 in a decidedly Cuban form. To see this process, it is necessary to bring into focus the concrete circumstance of public services. For the new system was launched with a surge of public health expansion from 1959 to 1961, which suggests that the implementation of the new system was a process of antagonism with both prerevolutionary and new revolutionary organization.

Aside from the familiar rural deficiency, the principal contradiction within the prerevolutionary government sector of health services had been the disparity between great formal centralization of authority, reaching directly from the national to the municipal level (without provincial or regional administration), and the separate and semiautonomous organization of operational units: dispensaries, first aid stations, general hospitals, and speciality factilities. The latter category included several lines of services (for example, for tuberculosis, venereal disease, leprosy, maternity, and pediatrics) which were administered by separate vertical agencies roughly under the direction of the ministry but often with appointment of officials directly by the president of the republic. Added to this inefficient structure (the more inefficient as optimal medical care became more expensive and complex) was a second contradiction, partially a product of the first: The always insufficient government funds, lost in graft and redundant administration, were unequaled by the even greater insufficiency of services provided. Since funds were always regarded as inadequate, administrators were said to have had few qualms for their misdirection. Since accountability was variable and distant from operations, few public servants experienced the constraints of personal accountability. For both of these reasons, the working conditions within the public sector were without the esprit de corps of internal cohesion and self-esteem, having neither social incentive nor social recognition.

It is into this structure that the new government poured investments after 1958 and where the expansion of rural services began as an independently administered sector. Unsurprisingly, one consequence of the burst of investment was to make old structural inefficiencies more costly and more apparent, while inexperienced administration and social disruption added new inefficiencies. To these rather simple difficulties of transition, one must add the similarly unsurprising inadequate planning of much rapid expansion in the absence of a clear methodology for rationalizing services or for the weighing of various needs. In this respect, it is extremely fortunate that the investments were generally directed by the rural priority. Here, as we have seen, there was a good plan for the organization of individual facilities, even if the notion of a rural network of services was yet immature. The rural focus meant, for the greater part, the building of primary facilities where the risk, for poor planning, was less than for conspicuous urban investments which had been the mark of the past (when the wife of each president felt compelled to found another hospital and each president a new plan for tuberculosis). In the delivery of a long needed rural service, nobody could quarrel with the first work of the revolution. By late 1961, however, shrinking resources and greatly expanded services meant that a simple approach to planning would no longer do. Great inefficiencies, over the long run, were possible. Isolated facilities were sometimes too elaborate for the low patient load and in relation to referral options. Sometimes locations were ill-chosen and, on occasion, too lux-urious. It was soon realized, for example, that too many small general hospitals were being built in rural areas.[41] Far more efficient in some cases than a rural hospital would have been the linkage of smaller, predominant-ly outpatient rural facilities with larger hospitals located in cities and large towns. That meant more and improved services for small urban centers.

One way or another the expansion of rural services was destined to place greater demands on the urban centers of rural regions. In this way, the rural emphasis on primary care, within a concept of comprehensive ser-vice, created its own politically influential pressure for a rationalized network of regional services. Just as more preventive services lead not to less but to greater demand for curative services, and more primary services raise demands for more secondary services, the expansion of rural services sharpened the previous contradiction between the simple level of rural and provincial services and the concentration of sophisticated services in the capital. That is, rural service pressured also for a national network of ser-vices. By building a base, attention was directed ultimately towards the system.

Working Out-of-Channels and Informal Organization

A sharp eye, dedicated to a complete view of the system under study here, would probably find very substantial informal and extrainstitutional developments that constituted real change in the health system that preceded (and also superseded) the formal structure reform of 1962. One would hypothesize that increased size in the absence of greater effective controls would lead to greater independence of far-flung units. New social programs and political mobilization would mean new relations between health facilities and the environment, and new patterns of social interaction that were not prescribed by the medical system proper. Clusters of services and personnel, with similar experiences, as in rural service, would likely lead to self-conscious interest groups.

A mechanical implementation of an external master plan, in the Cuban case, borrowing from the Czech model, was thus impossible. The plan, rather, would have to adapt itself to a vigorous mass of social activity, especially to the clusters of rural services with their own pressures for system rationalization from the bottom up. This would not have been the case if a new comprehensive state structure had been promulgated in early 1959.

Some of the variables involved in the hazy area of informal develop-ment would come to light in a careful study of organizational and ad-ministrative style. In fact, a new style might be reasonably considered one of the most important features of the new revolution. In a time when officials and health workers with operational responsibilities acted with great improvisation, a popular style of leadership was frequently seen which tended to involve everyone in decision making meetings. As at least one self-criticism has suggested, this style derived partly from technical incapacity and inexperience of new administrators[42] and also, one would suspect, from their ebullient good intentions. The transitional newness and imprecision of vertical lines of authority, and the absence of centralized norms for the internal administration of health facilities left wide degrees of freedom, which had the effect of shortening communication paths within organizations and opening channels among different organizations. These are characteristics which, of course, were manifest in other areas in an environment and mood which students of revolution may suggest are common to the aftermath of any successful and popular rebellion, or, to some extent, to young and growing organizations.[43] With boundless expectations, no difficulty seemed too great for revolutionaries to overcome, largely by being revolutionary, and new difficulties were easily created. The latter notwithstanding, the early period revealed energies that could be generated by moral and political exortation. Degrees of flexibility in health organization were tested, and leadership and organizational skills were developed.

If the Cuban rebellion had been an ordinary seizure of power, if external threats had been less extreme, if the pace of social change had not accelerated, and in the case of the health system, if the emigration of physicians had not been so pronounced, the period of the aftermath might have soon disappeared in the newly stabilized administration. As it was, the health system, like other social sectors, was kept in a state of flux.[44] To the disruption of the period was added the effects of the U.S. blockade, the nationalization of the large pharmaceutical firms in 1961, and the ban on the sale of a long list of medicinal products that were redundant or without medical quality.[45] Meetings necessarily turned into explanatory, pedagogical sessions, as much dedicated to external conditions as to the immediate internal problems of health organization. Threats of counter-revolution and sabotage led to the creation in 1960 of hospital vigilance committees, akin to the Committees for the Defense of the Revolution and the Vigilance and Public Health Committee of the Cuban Medical Federation.[46] The organization of the militia, the threat of invasion, and finally in 1962, the threat of nuclear war, involved physicians in emergency planning in collaboration with the army and other defense organizations. Many Cuban physicians and health workers were thus made aware of the grim implications of an invasion by the United States.

Such conditions magnified not only pressures for consensus and solidarity, but also as in the university, the social isolation of some. The high tide of this polarization in 1962 was marked, on the one hand, by the new plan for health organization and the antipolio campaign and, on the other hand, by the rather farfetched claims by disgruntled emigré physicians of deteriorating health and medical conditions.[47]

Creative Use of Task Forces or Groups

One may suppose that in such an arena of activity the simple declaration of new structural definitions, rules, and procedures would produce few substantial changes, the more certain since personnel were accustomed to working out of channels. But this was not the way that the substance of the new system was effected. The course of the new organization of services was set by the relationship of the ministry to practical matters. This relationship began in a flourish of technical activity under the initiative of the new Scientific Council of the ministry and the action programs in preventive medicine under the department of Hygiene and Epidemiology. Technical conferences were held on the regional, provincial, and national levels to establish norms or guidelines for many practical matters of health work and organization, and specific campaigns were planned.[48] Here, of course, the 1962 polio vaccination campaign was prototypical (and was repeated, with improvements, every year thereafter).[49] Norms and campaigns involved the formation of interspecialty and interorganizational task forces which were loosely attached to the vertical hierarchy established in 1962. Other practical directions included the organization in 1962 of a national chain of hospital libraries; guidelines and regulations for hospital administration; a plan for the evaluation of medical work with medical record review committees; and, along with the creation of residency specialization, the review by examination of all specialty credentials, thus finally ending the self-determination of specialists.

The creative role of this activity with respect to the internal organization of public health, rests, it seems to me, on the ability of these programs to follow informal networks to bring together the efforts of people from different institutions. This was facilitated because it was the cooperation of individuals rather than institutions that was initially involved, although, in the execution of consequent programs, institutional cooperation became the focus. Moreover, as activities that were functionally or professionally (rather than regionally or politically) defined, there was little conflict of hierarchy. At the same time it was easy to organize and channel such activities within the hierarchy defined by the new plan. Together these observations lend support to another: that the technical and scientific activities of the ministry served to create, through specific recruitment or cooptation (in the sociological sense), a vertically linked technical cadre under an increasingly prestigious national technical direction.[50] Indirectly, these activities also served to broaden the influence and practical exposure of university professors who inevitably were drawn into this activity.

This process is at once lubricant and cement; it raises the accessibility of vital information to all parts of a system while it creates extrainstitutional vertical bonds in an otherwise decentralized structure. It helped establish channels for a new system, and, as a special consequence of public health campaigns, it established channels for an active interface between

Diagram 6.2

Regional Direction of the Ministry of Public Health, 1962*

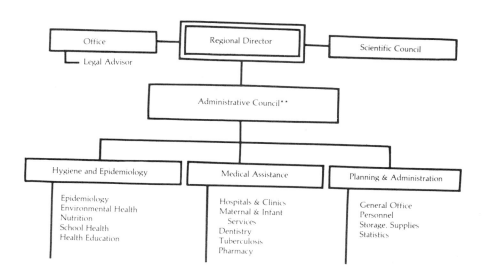

---

*Adapted from Cuba, Ministerio de Salud Pública, Subsecretaria de Economía. *Datos y cifras en salud pública, 1962*, Havana: Ministerio de Salud Pública, 1962.

**Members include the regional director and one representative each from Hygiene and Epidemiology, Medical Assistance, Planning & Administration, and the Scientific Council. Additionally, at least one representative of a regional facility is included.

health structures, other sectors, and community organizations.[51] Ties were formed between the new system and the conglomeration of informal networks that had already emerged in the first three or four years of public health work under the revolution.

MUTUALISM AND PRIVATE PRACTICE

As the history of Cuban mutualism unfolded in the 1950s, the distinctive contradiction had come to lie in the contrast between large and small mutualist programs. The principal difference between conditions of 1957 and those of 1934 was that older programs linked to Spanish immigration, had stabilized at a not greatly expanded size over the year 1934, while some of the newer programs, which were no longer really new, had expanded considerably.[52] Small mutualism continued to make wasteful use of physicians, whereas large programs continued to make wasteful use of hospital beds. While the ethnic exclusivity of older mutualism declined, ethnic conflict along Spanish-Cuban lines was hardly visible.[53] The leadership, however, of the still predominantly Spanish centers continued to be drawn from wealthy and politically conservative members. By contrast, the small program organized by the Transport Workers Union and leftist physicians in 1938 to have increased its size by 1957 and become a center of considerable experimentation and innovation, with emphasis on preventive medical efforts.[54] In sum, mutualism continued to be a significant, if essentially friendly, limiting constraint on private practice, tending to foster social approaches to health, illness, and medical care while, at the same time, helping to concentrate marginal physicians and services in urban areas. With regard to the latter, the 1959 provincial ratios of mutualist to public general hospital beds seems to relate to the cosmopolitanism of the province. Havana had a ratio (mutualist:public) of 72:34, compared to 7:11 in Camagüey and 4:14 in North Oriente. While mutualism covered perhaps half of Havana's population, it had more than twice as many general beds. Clearly, mutualism in Havana (and also, in relative terms, in other provinces as well) had many more physicians; for the all-Cuba 1962 ratio of physician to nurses (positions) was 34:44 in the public sector in comparison with 25:13 in mutualism.[55]

Private practice continued as small enclaves in virtually every public institution, always intensifying the pervasive second-class character of relatively free services to nonpaying patients.[56] This intrusion seems to have also increased within the units of mutualism. One form was the provision of unsalaried services by physcians in exchange for use privileges in the institution and accesss to private patients. This system, common everywhere in the United States, was known at an earlier time in Cuba, but was given greater encouragement after 1943 as a means of circumventing the regulation of minimum wage and single post that had been won by the Cuban Medical Federation. In spite of some achievements by the federation, a review of editorials in the *Tribuna Médica* during the 1950s strongly suggests that, while the CMC was busy negotiating a large number of individual cases, the same general problems remained; the old mutualist issues were often raised and the immobility of physicians was sometimes violated and constantly threatened.[57]

While revolutionaries had due cause to look askance at mutualism, mutualism continued to be the occasional target of conservatives. As late as October 1959, a physician, Enrique Ruiz Aguila, introduced the following unsuccessful motion at the National Medical Forum on Social Security, Mutualism, and Rural Medicine: "It is not logical that a country with a capitalist (democratic) system for the great majority, should have a socialist system for others (in this case mutualism in medicine), with all the undisputable disadvantages of socialist medicine, while it diminishes private medicine to a minimum."[58]

The new Ministry of Health began in 1959 with an ambivalent attitude toward mutualism, and, while the ministry was given the authority to demand the cooperation of all health-related institutions, it was slow to pressure drastic changes. A dual system emerged, then, with little public attention directed toward mutualist institutions. (Most of the few completely private nonmutualist clinics were nationalized by 1963; the most exclusive, a private hospital serving the wealthy Miramar suburb, became a special clinic for the many young scholarship students who soon occupied the abandoned mansions of the area.)

First Effects on Mutualism

Given the overburdened and second-class character of public facilities in prerevolutionary Cuba, the goal of most people who had to use public services was to achieve the economic status necessary to join a mutuality. Many even overextended their means, especially when they were pressured by salesmen who were retained by most mutualities. (Some representatives also collected the monthly fees, retaining an 8 to 10 percent commission.) If the economy did not decline, and certainly if personal income increased, such units would tend to grow.

One of the first consequences of the revolution for urban health services was an increase in mutualist membership. A substantial increase in disposable personal income was the immediate effect of the first measures of the revolution, notably the halving of urban rents and expansion of employment opportunities. While some poor persons now joined the religious sects of Santeria, paying upwards of one thousand dollars per initiation,[59] many other persons thronged to the membership rolls of mutualism. By 1966, mutualism may have included somewhat more than half of Havana's population and some 400,000 in other parts of Cuba. The latter figure was also influenced by the income redistribution policy and flow of resources to countryside, but the membership continued to be concentrated in a handful of interior cities, Santiago, Camagüey, Santa Clara, Matanzas, and Pinar del Río.[60]

What were the effects of these increases? First, they helped mitigate whatever effect the emigration of private physicians might have had on the general urban population. Second, they lessened certain pressures on public services as they underwent periods of reorganization. Third, the expansion increased the intensity of contradictions within mutualism, the increased numbers making more acute the consequences of "anarchy" among various services. The latter effect was strengthened by the limitation on physical and personnel expansion of mutualism that derived from two new external conditions. First, the aim of the new government was to expand and improve public facilities, with priority to new services in rural areas. Second, a general shortage of essential resources for health services developed in Cuba, at least after 1962 and 1963. Working together, these two conditions placed strong constraints on mutualism. The general condition was not altogether unlike the transformation of the Health Insurance Plan (HIP) of New York City, which underwent a rapid increase in membership at a time of skyrocketing medical costs. On the whole, these developments tended to reduce the disparities between mutualism and the public sector (the latter could expand, the former could not), but the intensification of problems within mutualism threatened to produce an antagonism between mutualism and the revolutionary government which seemed to be responsible for the painful constraints. A great achievement of the revolution was that it helped mutualism resolve the internal contradictions that were intensified, though not created, by the revolution itself.

The internal problems of mutualism took the form, first of all, that was described above. The inability of small mutualism to provide comprehensive services, often guaranteed on paper, was a more severe problem as membership increased. Under previous circumstances, this influx would have prompted a chaotic growth of duplicated services and facilities, an increase in the price of care, and a tendency to encourage, one way or another, more treatment under private arrangements within mutualism. Prohibited by government directives and by concrete circumstances in all of these directions, the directors and physicians of mutualism must have been frustrated indeed, restrained for the first time from acting in old ways. Not surprisingly, some eminent figures of mutualism retired from the country.

Resolution within Regionalization

Considering such problems, a task force on mutualism of the Ministry of Public Health was formed from mutualist physicians. Their report, presented in a national assembly of mutualism around 1963,[61] provided the basis for an official plan to consolidate and rationalize mutualism. The point of departure was the goal of achieving direct cooperation between large and small units. To this end, employing the principals of regionalization that were developing under the Czech model in the public sector, five

Diagram 6.3

Vertical Programs and Horizontal Cooperation

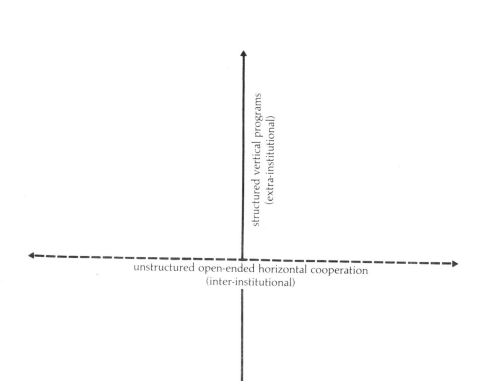

mutualist districts were created in Greater Havana, in each case assigning to the largest or most capable institution the role of base clinic. Each district collectively carried the obligation to arrange comprehensive health services for all its members, establishing necessary referral privileges, closing redundant or inefficient facilities, regrouping personnel, and expanding some services and facilties according to newly defined needs.

These measures eliminated the most glaring speculative nature of the pseudomutualities and financial irregularities that were known to exist even among the truly cooperative centers. Some private facilities, interestingly, were nationalized and incorporated into mutualist districts.

Psychiatric services provide an example of the process of regional integration. Although most mutualist plans included mention of psychiatric care, in reality only five large mutualities provided hospitalization (all elements, in fact, of "old" mutualism). With the exception of the women's quarters of Covadonga, no provision was made to separate acute cases from the much larger number of chronic cases, and thus, in the words of one writer, the hospitals "were converted into true warehouses of chronics." Hospitalization for men generally predominated while some care for women was contracted to a number of very small private clinics. Seven clinics provided irregular outpatient psychiatric consultations, not employing more than a few hours labor of one psychiatrist. Twenty-one clinics provided no psychiatric attention of any kind.[62] By 1965, however, regionalization provided a system which extended to all mutualist members hospitalization for all acute cases by referral, leaving the provision of outpatient services unresolved in only seven of Havana's mutualities. In this fashion, optimum use of scarce facilities and psychiatrists was achieved and psychiatric care was extended, with limitiations, to half of Havana's population and by referral to four hundred thousand *mutualizados* of other areas. Furthermore, since chronic care was greatly improved during the same period in the National Psychiatric Hospital,[63] it was reasonably intended that more hospitals would soon give greater attention to acute and chronic cases with potential for rehabilitation. In a related area, 15 private mental sanatoria, with a total of 816 beds, 299 for men and 517 for women,[64] were similarly studied and MINSAP intervened in various ways. Five were closed outright, it seems, for their "deplorable" state of services, one was closed for being too small, and one was converted to serve as the area health center for Guanabacoa. The remaining eight were combined in an administrative unit, roughly considered as a sixth district of mutualism. Finally, in 1966, 90 beds of one private hospital and the old Clínica La Bondad (a private general hospital with 175 beds) were dedicated to geriatric psychiatry, lessening the strain on other services. But humane treatment could be the only serious aim of such services, for all of these services employed the labor of only seven psychiatrists. These "mutualized" institutions incurred an obligation to accept referrals from mutualist clinics, especially from districts four and five which had no internal provision for hospitalization.[65]

Thus was built the basis for badly needed improvement in the quality of care. Medical care to mental patients was generally improved and a closer integration with general hospital services was urged. Work therapy, known as "ergotherapy" in Belgium, Holland, England, and the United States, was systematically begun, perhaps for the first time in Latin America. Statistical work, archives, and case review were systematized. In addition to making more efficient use of resources, the regionalized structure of mutualism made crystal clear the overall deficiencies and projected resource needs in psychiatric care, signaling the obligation of the medical school to train more and improved psychiatrists, psychiatric nurses, social workers, and trained auxilary personnel. The absence of health education measures and preventive orientations were also made apparent.

It may be concluded that, far from experiencing deterioration in the quality of care, the population of Havana, which was used to the irregular facilities of prerevolutionary mutualism, benefited in important ways from the early changes introduced under the revolution. The revolutionary Ministry of Public Health benefited, in turn, by experience and expertise that was developed within mutualism in the course of regionalization, and, more directly, by the growing cooperation between public and mutualist facilities.

NOTES

1. Ernesto (Ché) Guevara, "Visita del Comdte. Dr. Ernesto Guevara al Colegio Médico Nacional: Declaraciones del Dr. Guevara sobre la clase médica," *Tribuna Médica*, 20 (January-June 1959): 17.

2. Maurice Zeitlin, "Cuba: Revolution without a Blueprint," in Irving Louis Horowitz, ed., *Cuban Communism* (New Brunswick, N.J.: Transaction, 1970), pp. 81-92.

3. Cyrille Dechamp and Moisés Poblete Troncoso, *El problema médico y la asistencia mutualista en Cuba*, a report of the International Labor Office (Havana: no publisher indicated, 1934).

4. The themes of the conference are reported in the issues of the *Tribuna Médica* of that year and also in 1958. Anticipating the 1957 conference, the federation began work on a medical census and commissioned the eminent economist, Jacinto Torras, to prepare an economic study. See Jacinto Torras, "Los factores económicos en la crisis médica," *Economía y Desarrollo*, 3 (July-August 1973) 4: 7-33.

5. Yellow fever, a disease communicated by a domestic mosquito, was eliminated quickly; malaria, transmitted by a common marsh and field mosquito, was relegated to the countryside. Intestinal parasites were found in virtually the whole population of some rural areas, and typhoid fever, subject to prompt control, long continued as a disease of small towns and villages. Never achieving a complete registry of rural births, there was an abnormally high maternal mortality rate. See discussion, Commission on Cuban Affairs, *Problems of the New Cuba*, pp. 95-106.

6. Yet it was the famous clinician, Juan Santos Fernández, who as president of the Academy of Sciences was one of the first to speak against the cruel error of allowing the pastoral image of rural serenity to obscure the conditions of rural misery. See Juan Santos Fernández, "La Vida Rural," speech before the Academy of Sciences, May 19, 1915, *Cuadernos de Historia Sanitaria, no. 16*, (Havana: Ministerio de Salud Pública), 1965.

7. Capitalistic in the classical sense of the word, bent on the capitalization of clinics and hospitals where the productivity and division of labor could be increased and permit the owners (or controllers) to profit from the labor of other medical workers.

8. Thomas remarks, "The small towns of Cuba, without the charm of the big cities, nor the excitement, but also without immediate access to the country, were in many ways the most depressed parts of the island." (Thomas, p. 1095.) It was here, as in the poor makeshift suburbs of larger towns, that there was real hunger, rural people without land.

9. Commission on Cuban Affairs, *Problems of the New Cuba*, Wilson George Smillie, primary author of section on public health (New York: Foreign Policy Association, 1935), pp. 117-18, 121.

10. Drawing a sample from a nontown rural population of 2,500,000 in all of Cuba, the findings, as I interpret them, were as follows. With an average calorie intake of 2,500 (not counting sugar consumption), the diet on the day before the interview derived calories from the following: meat (4%), fish (less than 1%), eggs (2.12%), milk (11.22%), bread (3.36%), corn flour (7.0%), tubular root plants (22%), rice (24%), beans (23%), and green vegetables (0%). 43% could neither read nor write; 44% had never attended school. 82.6% had neither bath or shower; 88.5% used water from an outside well; 25% used an outside latrine (not a toilet); and 64% had no toilet provisions of any kind. With an average income of $45/month, 69.3% was spent on food, or $.25/day/person. Although only $2.00 (no base period given) were spent on medicines, the sources of medical assistance indicated were: private or *pago* (80.8%), public or free (8%), workplace or union (4%), private or mutualist dispensary (4%). 46.7% of homes had prescribed medicines. See Agrupación Católica Universitaria, "Encuesta de los trabajadores rurales, 1956-57," *Economía y Desarrollo*, 3 (July-August 1972) 12: 188-212.

11. Rafael Calvó Fonseca, Instituto Finlay, "Servicio de Salud en el Medio Rural: Proyecto de Organización Sanataria-Asistencial," *Revista KUBA* 15 (January-June 1959) 1-6: 8-15. The author was vice-president of the Medical Federation in 1946 after the victory of Acción Inmediata. (Fernández-Conde, p. 3.)

12. The Finlay Institute was a study and teaching unit jointly supported and oriented by the Ministry of Health and Social Assistance and the medical school. Its task was to guide and develop the public health career of physicians and to perform related research and teaching.

13. Calvó Fonseca, p. 9.

14. Ibid., p. 10.

15. See Manuel Amador García, Physician of the Rural Dispensary of Bernardo, Baracoa, Oriente, "Enfermedad y condiciones de vida" (presented at the 10th National Medical Congress), *Revista Cubana de Medicina* 2 (February 1963) 1: 34-45.

16. Carlos Font Pupo, "La salud del pueblo, preocupación básica de la Revolución," *Cuba Socialista* (April 1963): 57.

17. Ibid.

18. The analogy must be indicated between the experience of the rural physicians and the rural literacy volunteers in 1961. Indeed it was such experiences which welded the union between the "Moncada" and "post-Moncada" generations in Cuba. With unambiguous morality, the rural physicians were the counterpoint to the emigrating physicians of the same year. For an excellent discussion of generations, see Arlie Hochschild, "Student Power in Action," *Trans-action* 6 (April 1969) 6: 17-18. For an examination of rural-urban conflict in the role of the medical graduate in rural service, see Leopoldo Araujo Bernal, "Psicología Social: Un enfoque sobre sus límites y conceptos básicos," *Revista Cubana de Medicina* 4 (April 1965) 2: 129-36.

19. Amador García, p. 43. See also Eleuterio Mederos Torriente, post graduate in Rural Service, "El parasitismo intestinal en las montañas de Santa Catalina de Sagua de Tánamo" (presented at the 10th National Medical Congress), *Revista Cubana de Medicina* 2 (February 1963) 1: 57-62; and Manuel Michel Tressord and Orlando Robania, Polyclinic of the Zone of San Luis, "Parasitismo intestinal en la zona rural." Ibid., pp. 89-91.

20. Calvó Fonseca, p. 9. It is difficult to understate the effect of this imagery, made real by the marching of peasants into Havana in 1959.

21. Interview, 1969.

22. Juan M. Portuondo de Castro, *Como se apoderaron los comunistas de la Universidad de La Havana* (Miami: Ediciones del Directorio Magisterial Cubano (Exilio), n.d.), p. 42.

23. Ibid. See also chapter on education in Dudley Seers, ed., *Cuba: The Economic and Social Revolution* (Chapel Hill: University of North Carolina Press, 1964).

24. I owe a special opportunity of observation to my eminent colleagues at the Department of Sociology, The City College of the City University of New York, 1969-72.

25. See, e.g., Portuondo de Castro, p. 19.

26. This decorum was in many respects more nostalgic than real, especially following the outbreak of violent struggle between student groups after the occupation of the university by Batista's army in 1935. See Thomas, p. 700.

27. Portuondo de Castro, p. 19.

28. Ibid., p. 54.

29. The effect of departing numbers was considerably moderated by the absence of full-time faculty before 1959. New and usually quite competent faculty came from Latin America and socialist countries. Students returned from study abroad, while many were sent on foreign scholarships. With such help, and the teaching assistance of advanced students, the continuation of medical education was a difficult, but not impossible, task.

30. These were the students I met in Fall 1968. Students received free board, room, school supplies, and a monthly stipend depending on year and family status. For a discussion see Carlos Font Pupo, 1963.

31. Ministerio de Salud Pública, "Informe del Ministerio de Salud Pública a la XVII Asamblea Mundial de la Organización Mundial de Salud," *Cuba Socialista* 3 (June 1964) 3: 290.

32. "Relación de técnicos extranjeros que se encuentran contratado por el Ministerio de Salud Pública y la Junta Central de Planificación, 1964 y 1965," *Tribuna Médica*, 26 (January 1965-September 1966): 77-118.

33. See the last pages in de Lara.

34. See discussion, Carlos Font Pupo, 1963. Such a situation was unavoidable at a time of emigrating professionals, great practical urgency, and absence of clearly understood long-range perspective.

35. Luis Nájera, "Sobre la reforma de la enseñanza de la higiene y medicina preventiva en las facultivas de medicina," *Revista KUBA*, 10 (July-December 1954) 7-12: 42.

36. For discussion, see Leopoldo Araujo Bernal and Gloria Monteagudo, "Experiencia derivada de una práctica social realizada por alumnos de medicina," *Revista Cubana de Medicina* 5 (December 1966) 6: 673-84. Students worked in teams of four or five, with variable enthusiasm and success, complicated by other heavy demands of the medical curriculum. Student reports, reproduced in the article, are quite good.

37. Actually, given the circumstances of the time, the institute directed by the professors of that discipline at the university, was also their private property and carried their names Kourí-Basnuevo. A subsidiary pharmaceutical enterprise Laboratorios KUBA, S.A. helped to finance and in turn be advertised by the journal of the Institute, the *Revista KUBA*. A history of parasitology and tropical medicine in Cuba may be found in Virgilio Beato Núñez, "Historia de la parasitología y de la medicina tropical en Cuba," *Revista KUBA* 4 (1948) 1:10-21. Interestingly, the courses in this subject were founded by the university reforms of 1923.

38. The prerevolutionary pharmaceutical industry reflected the disposition of health services: more than 250 small laboratories (but a total of 500 producers) alongside some 14 larger and better equipped installations. With little technical control of 30,000-40,000 products, only 4,000 were recognized and subject to supervision of the pharmaceutical council of the Colegio Médico. 2,223 pharmacies were registered in 1958, following the same extreme patterns of concentration around neighborhoods of greater wealth. Decree No. 709 of March 23, 1959, reduced the prices of domestic products by 15% and imported products by 20%. Political events preceded the nationalization of pharmaceutical firms. Reminiscent of Romay's directive of 1842, only 1,000 of the 4,000 ethical products were found essential to modern therapy; laboratories were closed, equipment and facilities were centralized, although not without creating difficulties and various disruptions (to which were added the consequences, still in force today, of the U.S. blockade and embargo). Rural pharmacies were created as urban pharmacies were nationalized after 1962. While more than 200 drugs were placed under rigid prescription, the number of urban pharmacies between 1958 and 1968 decreased from 2,200 to 960; rural pharmacies increased from 60 to 305; and pharmacies in Vedado decreased from 102 to 28. See analysis, Ministerio de Salud Pública, *Diez Años de Salud Pública* (Havana: Instituto del Libro, 1969, pp. 141-54).

39. When Cuban physicians studied health services in several countries, the Czech system was understandably impressive. A few years after the almost complete destruction of health facilities, the loss of nearly half of the country's physicians in World War II, and transition to socialism, organized health services existed for even the most remote village and were linked, in a comprehensive regionalized system of personal and environmental, curative and preventive activities, to sophisticated centers of medical research and practice. Besides, the Czechs, who in 1960 had vaccinated 93% of all children under fifteen against polio, offered to assist Cuba in conducting a similar campaign, complete with free Sabin vaccine manufactured in the Soviet Union. See the following: Milton I. Roemer, "World Trends in Medical Care Organization," *Social Research* 26 (Autumn 1959) 2: 283-310, es-

pecially 294-95; Weinerman, *Social Medicine in Eastern Europe*, especially pp. 46-87; and Dr. Stich, Vice Minister of Public Health of Czechoslavakia, "Coordinación e integración de los servicios de Salubridad en Czechoslavakia" (presented at the Tenth National Medical Congress, Havana, February 17-24, 1963), *Revista Cubana de Medicina* 3 (June 1964) 3: 354-60.

40. Personal interviews, Ministry of Public Health, 1968.

41. Carlos Font Pupo, "Hacia la salud pública socialista," *Cuba Socialista* (July 1965). This article by Font Pupo signals the change in attitude from that expressed in his earlier (1963) article on the same subject.

42. See, e.g. Luis Rodríguez Rivera, "Métodos de dirección colectiva en nuestra actual organización hospitalaria," *Revista Cubana de Medicina* 3 (August 1964) 4: 388.

43. Wilensky, *Organizational Intelligence*, ch. i.

44. One of the most valuable views of the inside of this process is given in Edward Boorstein, *The Economic Transformation of Cuba* (New York: Monthly Review Press, 1968).

45. See note no. 34 above. The close relations between legitimate medicine and the commerce in useless or deceptive medicines is recorded in the advertisements which appear in almost every prerevolutionary medical journal.

46. It is possible that this committee was a continuation of (or a confusion with) a committee of the Havana Medical College that existed already in 1957, whose aim was to check the widespread unrestricted sale of prescription medicines. See editorial, "Salus Populus," *Boletín del Colegio Médico de La Habana* 8 (April-May 1957) 4-5: 145-46.

47. See, for example the reply to one accusation, Luis Gómez Wangüemert, "Falsedad Desmentida," *Revista Cubana de Pediatría* 34 (September-October 1962) 5: 1-2.

48. Campaigns were planned against gastroeneritis, malaria, tuberculosis, and leprosy. Norms were developed for statistical records, administration of obstetric services, hospital care of newborn babies and their mothers, and pediatric vaccinations.

49. Carried out amid a peak of polarizing political tendencies and great public fanfare, the socialist organization of health services and concept of preventive medicine was launched with the most impressive public health event since the eradication of yellow fever.

50. These vertically organized technical cadres continue to play an important but recently diminishing role today. See discussion by Vicente Navarro, "Health, Health Services, and Health Planning in Cuba," *International Journal of Health Services* 2 (August 1972) 3: 397-432. Navarro's article (the most complete and well-informed analysis of contemporary organization of Cuban health care) suggests that the vertical organizations, which have grown in number, may be leading in 1971 to new organizational problems of coordination between separate *disease* (rather than functional) orientations. Not to overstate the role of interinstitutional structures, perhaps of equal importance was the establishment, by departmentalization, of norms of collective administration of health services. Of this subject, an excellent discussion is that of Luis Rodríguez Rivera. See note 41, above.

51. The Committees for the Defense of the Revolution were formed, mostly spontaneously, in 1960 to prevent counterrevolutionary activities. Soon integrated in public health efforts, they early constituted a very real community voice and participation in health matters.

52. The number of private clinics seems also to have expanded, for in 1958 there were a total of 242 private or mutualist clinics with more than ten permanent beds compared with 97 public hospitals; 94 clinics were in Havana alone. The most definitive work in the subject of hospital development is Francisco Rojas Ochoa, Director, Planning and Statistics Group, Ministry of Public Health, "La red hospitalaria del Ministerio de Salud Pública en el período 1958-1969," *Revista Cubana de Medicina* 10 (January-February 1971) 1: 3-42.

53. See Thomas, pp. 180-83.

54. See Carlos Font Pupo, "Quinta Reunión anual y extraordinaria del Cuerpo Médico del Centro Benéfico Jurídico de Trabajadores de Cuba, palabras del Dr. Carlos Font Pupo, Director de la Clínica, en la Aperatura del Acto," *Boletín del Colegio Médico de La Habana* 8 (April-May 1957) 4-5: 148-51.

55. Cuba, Ministerio de Salud Pública, Subsecretaria de Economía, pp. 51 and 60.

56. One statesman of presocialist medicine complained, for example, that medical students treated the aged public patients of Calixto García without the respect that should be accorded to any older person. "On top of the triple misfortune of being poor, ill, and having to be in Calixto García, the aged poor were then made to feel like dirt." (Interview, 1969). In the absence of qualitative studies of immediately prerevolutionary health care, perhaps the best description is by analogy with the similar, but probably more severe, chaos that characterizes the contemporary system in Argentina. See, in this regard, Jorge Segovia and Omar J. Gómez, "Implicit vs. Explicit Goals: Medical Care in Argentina" draft of an article to be published in Stan Ingman and Anthony Thomas eds., *Topias and Utopias in Health* (The Hague: Mouton, 1974).

57. See the editorial, "El Médico en las Instituciones Benéficas," *Boletín del Colegio Médico de La Habana* 8 (March 1957) 3: 107.

58. "Forum Médico National Sobre Seguridad Social-Mutualismo y Medicina Rural (octubre 30-31, noviembre 1ro, 1959)," archives of the Cuban Medical Federation, Havana: Museo de la Historia de las Ciencias "Carlos J. Finlay." One of the chief controversies of this conference had to do with the government's contemplated consolidation of the more than twenty different retirement and accident insurance funds. Many physicians did not want their funds administered with workers' social security funds. But in 1961, the funds were not only consolidated but placed under the Ministry of Labor for administration. Technical data are found in Oficina Internacional del Trabajo, *Informe al Gobierno de Cuba sobre seguridad social*, Geneva: International Labor Office, 1960 (mimeographed).

59. Interview, Museum of Afro-Cuban Culture, Regla, 1968.

60. This is suggested by the scarce provision of psychiatric assistance in mutualism, available only in these cities outside of Havana. See Jorge López Valdés, "Organización de la asistencia psiquiátrica en el mutualismo," *Revista Cubana de Medicina* 5 (January-Febuary 1966) 1: 80.

61. The date is my guess from imperfect notes of interviews, 1968.

62. Five of them were closed; others were merged or changed function. Ibid., pp. 68-69.

63. The National Psychiatric Hospital has become a showplace of humanist efforts by the revolutionary government. Its work expanded until 1965, when efforts were begun to build two other hospitals for chronic patients, while acute care is being integrated into the general hospital system. The background is provided by

a history of cruel and graft-ridden administration, dating to the degradation in the same institution (as early as 1879) of aged and incapacitated slaves.

64. López Valdés, pp. 68-69.

65. This seems implicit in López Valdés.

7
Consolidation of a Comprehensive National System

AREA POLYCLINIC

At this point, the writing of history merges with an analysis of the contemporary system. This means, in the Cuban case, an analysis of the evolving role of the area polyclinic, Cuba's community health center. Faced with a growing bottleneck in the delivery of ambulatory services, a problem which sprang from the direction and velocity of the early transformations, a decision in 1965 established the area polyclinic as the point of departure for all health planning. This focus has been maintained in the ensuing years, and, indeed, the intensity of this institutional focus is so pronounced that a detailed examination of the area polyclinic goes a long way toward describing the health system itself. Moreover, the development of the area polyclinic has strongly influenced, and is paralleled by, developments in other spheres, in particular the training of physicians and other health workers.

The area polyclinic was not invented in 1965, but its general form and expanded future role were decided. This decision was pressured as I have just suggested, by practical problems that arose in the first five years of revolution. But as previous discussion suggests, the roots of invention and Cuban predisposition for the polyclinic lay elsewhere: in the rural health center, mutualist organization, dispensaries of the prerevolutionary ministry of health, and Czechoslovakian experience. When to these preconditions are added the political disdain for private practice as a vestige of capitalism and the technical disdain for the sole office practitioner and small clinic as archaic forms of health services delivery, the new Cuban polyclinic seems to follow as if by logic.

163

Considering the closeness of the period which is now under discussion (1965-1971), much of what will be said in the fashion of system description remains valid today. Indeed, it is fairly safe to presume that most descriptive statements which are not somehow amended in the discussion of the next period continue to apply. I will, however, continue to use the past tense, for I want to give proper credit to the distinctiveness of the period discussed, and I wish to avoid the appearance of making an exaggerated claim to having described the present reality, which, of course, has its own dynamics of change.

Rationalization and the Problem of Ambulatory Care

The first years of the revolution led to new gaps, as well as improvements in health services. Rationalization of health services motivated, for example, the closing of many small, mostly urban hospitals and the expansion of others. As in other countries in the same period, but exacerbated in Cuba by the unique international disruption of resources, it was increasingly difficult (due partly to technological changes requiring greater specialization and supportive facilities) for small hospitals, say under 100 beds, to efficiently provide the range of services that had come to be expected of a general hospital. A 1971 report on the Cuban health system reveals surprising statistics on this process. 63 percent of hospital beds existent in 1969 were new after 1958, but there was a decrease from 339 to 219 in the number of "hospitals," while the average number of beds rose from 83 to 181, and the number of hospital beds increased from 25,170 to 41,027, or in per capita terms, from 3.8 to 5.1 beds per 1,000 inhabitants.[1]

In the same period, the large increase in public employment of physicians, and the flight of physicians from the country, were two sides of a process which drew physicians from other categories, from private and mutualist practice. The magnitude of this process is suggested by its outcome. *By 1970, only 600 of Cuba's 7,000 physicians were in private practice, and, of these, only 80 were engaged full-time. Most were older physicians of Havana.*[2]

New Bottleneck of Services

The concentration and growth of large hospital services, which by 1965 were better distributed[3] throughout the country, and the diminution of private office, private clinic and mutualist practice[4] together contributed to a bourgeoning demand for the outpatient services of large hospitals. This was consistent with the establishment, in 1962 and 1963, of provincial and regional administrations and service levels on the Czech model. Yet by 1965, amid visibly improved and expanded hospital, environmental, and preventive medical services, a crisis was approaching in the provision of continuous outpatient services. More services were being rendered, but with visible inconvenience, travel, and waiting periods for patients. When, for example, the magnificently modern and well-equipped Lenin Hospital of Holguín opened in 1962 as the provincial hospital center of North Oriente, an avalanche of patients descended upon the new Mecca. Where services were previously lacking, the new bottleneck in follow-up and continuity of care threatened to weaken the contribution of new hospital investment. As previous patterns of care were disrupted, the first tendency was to increase demands on the outpatient services of public hospitals.[5]

Inevitably, some argued that resources would be better spent on smaller and, perhaps, less efficient hospitals, or on small outpatient clinics. (Elsewhere, of course, experts were arguing that preventive and environmental services should be emphasized in poor nations, to the *abandonment* of extensive clinical efforts.)[6] A dilemma of services, then, paralleled the conflict between the activities which were begun before 1962 and the rationalization of services within the Czech model. The former had emphasized the extension of small units in the rural periphery and the consolidation of prerevolutionary services; the latter increased the concentrated organization, from the top down, of hospital and specialist services.

The Cuban Solution

The resolution of these tensions was moderated by two commitments: (1) a commitment against the substitution of nonphysicians for physicians in the delivery of primary care and (2) a commitment to the eventual integration of all primary services with the most sophisticated hospital care. The emigration of physicians made the first commitment a matter of national pride. The second, given the level of prerevolutionary services in Havana, was supported by the overall commitment of the revolution to egalitarian values. Both commitments were strongly supported by the great influence of physicians in the determination of technical orientations.

The concrete development, argued by all of the above, was a decision in 1965 by the Ministry of Public Health to establish and emphasize the polyclinic and the "health area" as the basic Cuban unit of health services delivery and administration. While larger hospital units continued to be the central trend of hospital organization, the polyclinic — *predominantly an outpatient facility independent of hospital control* — was regarded as the core of the health services system as a whole. This decision institutionalized the independence of two contrary directions of expansion within a creative relationship, the "centralization of inpatient services and the decentralization of outpatient services."[7]

HEALTH SYSTEM

Regionalization

It will be helpful, before completing the examination of the area polyclinic, to cast a glance at the larger system. By 1967, virtually all professional services related to health were incorporated within the Ministry of Public Health (MINSAP), and the components of this consolidated system interrelated within a logic of regionalization. In such a comprehensively socialized system of health services, some fashion of identity exists between each organizationally defined enterprise of health promotion and some sociodemographic region. The Cuban model circa 1968-1972 (see Diagram 7.1) identified four levels of regionalization: area, region, province, and nation. This set of organizational levels constitutes a hierarchy of backup services, resource networks, planning capabilities, and mechanisms of coordination. Additionally, each level was consciously designed as a nexus of interaction between the health system and the social environment.

Diagram 7.1
The Cuban Health System—Four Pillars and
Levels of Health Promotion

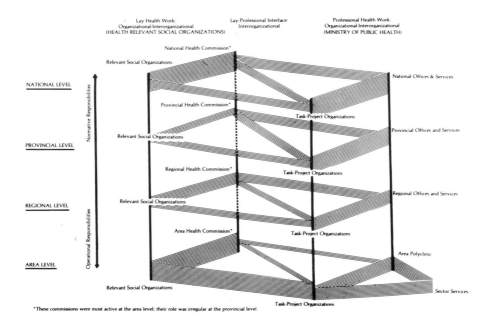

Within the constraints of historical legacy (institutional concentration in Havana, in particular) and various practical considerations, the location of service and responsibility was indicated by the slogan adopted in the 1963 plan, "normative centralization and administrative decentralization." To illustrate, by reference to categories of physician services, the area polyclinic guaranteed the spectrum of primary services in an ambulatory setting; provided somewhat variable access to secondary specialties, also on an ambulatory basis; and guided the patient to the appropriate hospital and specialty services that were provided in regional[8] and provincial settings. Direct responsibility for hospital and physician services was minimized at the national level, rendering the provincial level the practical apex of services. The principal functions of the national level were normative and budgetary. In addition, the national level was developing direct responsibility for the service, research, and teaching functions of ten national institutes, three medical schools (although here the primary administrative authority continued to be with the Ministry of Education), various training programs for technical personnel, and postgraduate training of physicians.

Interorganizations and Community Interface

A continuing feature of the Cuban system was an increasingly institutionalized role for specialized, task-oriented national organizations. Disease or problem-specific campaigns (for example, cancer detection for women) and technical committees, groups or task forces on medical-sanitary procedural norms (for example, postpartum care) predominate. With open, semistructured horizontal components and structured vertical components, such organizations served, I think, as an important kind of organizational glue for the early emerging system. (However, in the course of this period, such benefits were increasingly measured against problems of redundant vertical parallelism and overemphasis on disease and problem categories.)[9]

One feature of these coordinative, project-defined structures was that they effectively incorporated the collaboration of lay groups and institutions. This lay-professional or society-health system interface was also, and most importantly, structured within a hierarchy of public health commissions, standing committees established at different organizational levels to effect interorganizational coordination and evaluate planning output. These commissions were key units of the health system but, significantly, they were not part of the ministry itself. Indeed, the health commissions were considered to have formal authority over the corresponding hierarchical levels of the ministry.

The interaction between the community and the health system suggests two perspectives, which I will develop in the following two sections, for examining the area polyclinic which evolved between 1969 and 1970.

First, I will examine the area polyclinic as a unit which looks inward toward the health system; and, second, as a unit which looks outward to the community. (See Diagram 7.2.) In part, this is a real division, for there is a real tension between the two perspectives; but it is also an abstract distinction which violates the unitary identity of the area polyclinic as the health system of the community.

Diagram 7.2
The Area Polyclinic in Cuban Society

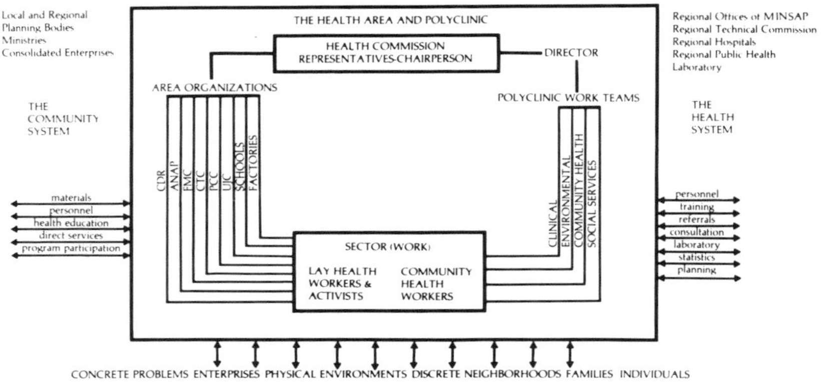

POLYCLINIC IN THE HEALTH SYSTEM

The polyclinic was designed to provide, integrate, or otherwise be responsible for the provision of four health functions — clinical services, environmental services, community health services, and related social services — to a specifically defined area and population. Under the leadership of a physician-director, these functions were served by four health teams. With an average population of 25,000 (in one instance, 60,000) in urban areas and sometimes as few as 7,500 in rural areas, the health areas were intended to be small enough to be accessible and large enough to efficiently provide a substantial range of primary services. These primary services included the typical "public health" tasks of sanitary control and community health work, organized and directed from the same organization that provided clinical and social services. *Thus, the goal, predominant in all socialist societies, of integrating curative-preventive and clinical-social-environmental dimensions was served in Cuba by the central role of the polyclinic.*

Administrative Independence

As the principal point of entry to the health system, it became the task of the polyclinic to define, orient, and protect the relationship of the health area population to the system of hospital and specialist services. To foster such a relationship, Cuban health leaders determined that the polyclinic should enjoy administrative independence from the hospital. Unlike similar institutions in other countries, including Czechoslovakia, the most directly relevant socialist prototype, the Cuban polyclinic was not to be an administrative extension of a regional hospital but was, like the regional hospital, an administrative unit under the purview of the regional office of the Ministry of Public Health. It was with the plans, problems, and proposals of the health areas, on the one hand, and of the regional services on the other, that health plans were composed at the regional level, the bottom and increasingly most important level in the formal process of Cuban health planning.

Independence, however, does not imply isolation. The polyclinic director was a member, alongside other health officials, of the regional technical committee which elaborated the primary operative component of national health planning. Hospitals and other health organizations, laboratories and epidemiological services were charged with specific obligations to the polyclinic. While each polyclinic employed a core of full-time staff, hospital physicians were required to work part-time in nearby polyclinics, providing primary services and specialist consultation. This measure was intended to encourage a community focus by hospital-based specialists. On the polyclinic side, staff physicians were required, whenever possible, to serve for short periods in the regional or provincial hospitals. This requirement was facilitated, indeed the whole relation between polyclinic and hospital is facilitated, by the policy of training primary care specialists rather than comprehensive generalists.

Thus, the clinical team of the polyclinic included, in 1968-1971, physicians and nurses working in internal medicine, pediatrics, obstetrics-gynecology, and dentistry, with primary care specialists who were available, on a part-time basis, from the staffs of nearby hospitals. In addition, many general practitioners moved from their solo office to the polyclinic where they continued to provide traditional general services. Nurses, it seems under this arrangement of organized primary services, began to assume greater clinical responsibilities, a tendency which showed signs of resolving some of the unsettled questions of the nursing profession.[10] The polyclinic, then, in Cuba replaced the general practitioner (and comparable roles in private and mutualist clinics), but the core staff of the polyclinic consisted of primary care *specialists*, nurses, and auxiliary personnel.

Staffing and Supplies

The breadth of responsibility in health matters is suggested by the categories of personnel in the polyclinic.

Table 7.1

Minimal Personnel Norms for the Area Polyclinic, 1971*

Personnel Categories	Number of Hours/Population Ratios
Director	1 full-time for each polyclinic
Internist	4 hours/day/15,000 people
Pediatrician	4 hours/day/3,000 children, ages 0-14
Obstetrician-gynecologist	4 hours/day/20,000 women
Dentist	8 hours/day/7,000 people
Dental assistant	1 full-time for each 15 dentist hours
Nurses	1 full-time for each polyclinic
Auxiliary nurses	1 for each sector (3,000-5,000 people)
Administrator	1 full-time for each polyclinic
Statistical clerk	1 full-time for each polyclinic
Laboratory technician	8 hours/day/15,000 people
Auxiliary technical sanitarian	1 full-time for two sectors
Assistant technical sanitarian	1 full-time for 2,000 people

*Source: V. Navarro, "Health, Health Services, and Health Planning in Cuba," *International Journal of Health Services* 2 (August 1972):409-10.

The above personnel, in Table 7.1 together with unclassified workers, were responsible for eight programs: maternal and child care, adult medical care, dentistry, control of infectious diseases, environmental services, food control, school health services, and occupational and labor medicine. In 1971, the principal staffing shortages were for dentists, dental assistants, and auxiliary technical sanitarians. National norms, the above source also reports, were often exceeded in other categories.

With regard to the match between patient demand and availability of services in the polyclinic, progress is probably indicated between 1968 and 1970. In 1968, I found some crowded waiting rooms and occasional reference to this phenomenon by Cuban physicians. Observers in 1970 and 1972, however, not only found polyclinics uniformly staffed at levels consistent with national norms, but also found waiting rooms well-managed and uncrowded.[11] While total outpatient visits to all categories of institutions almost doubled from 1964 to 1969, the percentage of such visits to general hospitals declined, from 28 percent to 19 percent. Percentages for polyclinic visits increased from 32 percent to 63 percent of all visits. Rural hospitals, with 6.1 percent of outpatient visits in 1965, accounted for only 3.2 percent in 1969 (although without greatly reduced absolute numbers).[12] Such statistics reflect decreases in private and mutualist practice, an increase in the number of polyclinics (192 to 289 in the same period), and growing familiarity with their role by the general population.[13] Appointments were recommended but not required, and one could usually be attended to at any polyclinic or outpatient facility. However, after a first visit, the patient is urged to go next to the polyclinic associated with his residence.

All services and medicines which were administered in polyclinics and hospitals were provided free of charge. Medicines purchased in pharmacies were sold at nominal prices and certain medicines, such as insulin, that were chronically required by the patient were either freely provided or provided at very reduced price. Pharmacies, which had been rationalized after their nationalization in 1963[14] were made directly responsible to the area polyclinic, while their supply and technical direction fell wholly under the purview of MINSAP.

POLYCLINIC IN THE COMMUNITY

The polyclinic in the community was manifested in two kinds of roles: the role of community health workers in local neighborhoods and the role of the polyclinic director as chairperson of the area health commission.

Local Neighborhood Organization

The direct neighborhood work was organized geographically into neighborhood health sectors, with a growing national average of 8.3 sectors per area.[15] To each sector the polyclinic sought to assign a field nurse, a sanitarian, and, sometimes, a social worker. In addition to the unsurprising tasks of such personnel, it is through them that technical support was given and collaboration is maintained with the extensive health-related functions of lay neighborhood organizations. Depending on geographical conditions, first aid posts could also be found in the sector, staffed by volunteers, auxiliary nurses, and, especially in rural areas, by teachers. Significant numbers of auxiliary personnel, as well as nontechnical volunteers, were also recruited from folk practitioners who were judged capable of enlarging their technical capacity. This was more the practice in rural areas where, for example, more than one thousand folk midwives were counted before 1962 in South Oriente alone.[16]

Unlike Eastern European countries, the Cuban Red Cross was dwarfed in importance beside the voluntary health work of the mass organizations. Only in the countryside were Red Cross first aid stations developed under that name, frequently staffed by rural teachers. However, since 1969, the Ministry of Public Health and the mass organizations began to experiment with the Red Cross as a means of achieving greater institutionalization in the role of voluntary health workers at the level of health sector, or neighborhood level. According to one plan that was partially carried out in spring 1969, one Red Cross operative would work full-time in each polyclinic and, with the collaboration of community health workers, he would coordinate the effort of perhaps thirty volunteers in each sector. Volunteers would staff first aid stations and ambulance services.[17] In addition to regular provision of very important services (in a country of rising accident rates), it was thought that such a plan could help to reduce redundancy among voluntary health workers on the neighborhood level and free the technical staff of the polyclinic from many organizational tasks. Perhaps, I thought, after learning of this experiment, the Red Cross station and the Red Cross operative of the polyclinic might someday function on the level of the sector as the Health Commission did on the level of the area. Any development along such lines would be of special interest to those who have tended to explain the surprisingly large role of voluntarism in Cuba by simple reference to the newness of the socialist system.

In any event, in 1968, Cuban health leaders spoke of the consolidation of the sector as a final stage of structural development. I hypothesized, therefore, in my 1972 manuscript that it may be at the level of the sector that one might expect new roles to evolve which might complement the somewhat impersonal and discontinuous tendencies of medical care in the polyclinic, which derive from mobility of personnel, part-time appointments, heavy patient loads or, in some urban cases, large size.[18]

Public Health Commissions

Considering that the polio campaign and other health work by lay groups antedate the formal organization of the sector and the health area, it is clear that the motivation and orientation for such work has strong origins that are independent of the Ministry of Public Health. The coordination and technical orientation of this energy were institutionalized at various levels after 1962 in the horizontal structures that have come to be known as "public health commissions." Because such cooperation was largely related to immediate problems of area and region, and to plan execution rather than formal plan preparation (the latter, especially its normative elements, tended to be centralized at the national and provincial levels), the area and regional commissions, in that order, developed the greatest vitality. But while provincial commissions were either eliminated or lived a sporadic existence, a National Health Commission actively assisted in the formulation of national health plans and in the development of national norms for the health activities of revolutionary organizations.

The Area Health Commission often included representatives from the following organizations:

1. *The Committees for the Defense of the Revolution* (CDR) were organized on the neighborhood and block level in 1960 to guard

against sabotage and to assist in the organization of the militia. After 1960, the organization broadened its activities in support of all manner of mobilization, especially for voluntary work in agriculture and for public health tasks. After 1962, the CDR was given virtually complete responsiblity for polio immunization and kept a record of other immunization schedules for special risk persons in the local neighborhood. With an estimated 1968 membership of over one-third of the population, the CDR is easily the most important mass organization in Cuba.[19]

2. *Poder Local* was an administrative council, a kind of local government, whose officials were elected, sometimes with great fanfare, by the CDR's under the guidance of the Communist Party. It seems to have been chiefly concerned with physical planning and maintenance, water supply, sewage and waste disposal, street repair, and the like. Its exact powers or methods of election or appointment to office were varied and often unclear. (Its functions are replaced today by elected government assemblies.)

3. *National Association of Small Farmers* (ANAP) was created to serve the interests of small farmers who remained or became established in the private sector of agriculture in the two early programs of agrarian reform in 1959 and 1960. It was perhaps the first mass organization to assist the work of early rural health centers.

4. *The Federation of Cuban Women* (FMC), like the CDR, is a mass organization with a national hierarchy of committees, from local to national level. Unlike the CDR, however, the FMC was created more from the top down than from the bottom up. Its influence has been bolstered by the prominent role of women who played a highly visible role in the liberation struggle. Assisted by liaison with the CDR, the FMC extended its base and has played an important role in health education activities, pediatric attention, maternal health, and family nutrition. In 1972 it assisted in a national study of child development which is, perhaps, the most complete study of its kind.

5. *The Confederation of Cuban Workers* (CTC) dates from prerevolutionary days. Its early communist leadership was purged after World War II by the Orthodoxo government of Carlos Prío Socarrás and his anticommunist strongman, Eusebio Mujal, who continued his role, unchanged under Batista. With the defeat of anticommunist tendencies in 1959, the CTC has gradually taken on the role of critical partnership with revolutionary management of socialized production. It is through the CTC that safety committees and first aid stations are organized in factories and state farms.

6. *The Cuban Communist Party* (PCC) was formed in 1965 from the

United Party of the Socialist Revolution (PURS) which had, in turn, been formed in 1961-62 from the Integrated Revolutionary Organizations (ORI). The latter included several groups, some of which ceased separate formal existence in 1962 and the most predominant, The Partido Socialista Popular (PSP — the old communist party) and the 26th of July Movement ceased separate formal existence in 1965. PCC members are selected for their exemplary qualities as workers and revolutionaries, which means among other things, that they must be well liked, stand out in voluntary efforts, and show qualities of leadership. As communists, they are expected to improve their political formation, which means that they must understand the economic plans and problems of Cuba and the communist goals of development. Materials of political education for party cadre will more likely be the highly substantive speeches of Fidel Castro or technical literature, than the writings of either Marx or Lenin. Concretely, party members serve as general trouble shooters; when people or organizations are not functioning or coordinating, it is the task of the party and its members to orient others in seeking a solution to inefficiency, conflict, or problem. The highest body is a Central or National Committee of one hundred members, and its executive committees. Under the Central Committee have slowly been established provincial and regional committees and base committees in the work place, where new members enter the party. (The role of the party was more clearly defined by the Socialist Constitution in 1975.)

7. *The Union of Young Communists* (UJC), like the Communist Party, is a cadre or vanguard organization, with a structure similar to the Communist Party itself. Its role too is similar, but focuses more on the matters that relate to young people, under twenty-five years of age. It is especially active among the various federations of secondary and university students and in the various "youth columns" and work brigades of young people, as for example on the Isle of Youth, formerly the Isle of Pines.

All of the above organizations included certain members who took special interest and responsibility in matters relating to health, and, as such, were known as *responsables de salud*. They were not, however, mechanically included on every health commission. ANAP was more important than the CDR and the CTC in some rural areas. Sometimes the Communist Party and Young Communists attended meetings by invitation rather than by regular attendance, and the attendance at many meetings appeared to be determined by the specific problem under discussion. An unusual problem focus or special characteristics of an area also invited participation by other health specialists and representatives of key organizations: factory managers, farm administrators, school or hospital officials, and so forth. Some commissions, especially in urban areas, met regularly, every two weeks, to review health conditions and health efforts; other commissions met irregularly, which perhaps helped to secure a problem orientation against ritualized agenda. It was through the health commissions (but not restricted to them, or to other formal channels) that a variety of citizen views, complaints, criticism, and ideas were effectively impressed upon the health personnel who shape the conduct of health work and planning.[20]

The influence on the public health commissions of lay organizations, and of the mass organizations in particular was neither a simple consequence of the commission itself nor of the political maxim which favored popular participation, although these factors lended significant structure and orientation. *The influence of lay organizations derived from their strong political footing in Cuban socialism and especially from their record of accomplishments and continuing responsibilities in health efforts,* beginning with the polio vaccination campaign of 1962. Since that date, the CDR had taken virtually complete administrative responsibility for polio vaccination and, in collaboration with the FMC, kept an up-to-date census of children, mothers, and pregnancy, along with their respective schedules of immunization and medical visits. It was also the task of the CDR to secure the registration of the entire population at their respective polyclinic. The CTC secured regular medical examinations for workers in the food service industries, health centers, and hospitals; and also assisted in the preparation and enforcement of sanitary work norms. ANAP collaborated in the control of animal brucelosis and tuberculosis; and the FMC organized examinations for early detection of cancer in women. Health education was undertaken with initiative by all mass organizations. A very popular form was the *audiencia sanitaria*, a health seminar which invited speakers from all ranks of health professionals. The CDR yearly celebrates the eve of its anniversary by holding a celebration in Havana that featured an address by the Minister of Public Health and was followed by outdoor health seminars along one of Havana's principle avenues.

A Socially Influential Institution

When the Health Commission was assembled, in 1968, it was thought to be the most widely representative body of its kind in Cuba. Other ministries and enterprises assembled similar, but less representative commissions to gain cooperation and participation on other fronts of the revolution. In fall 1968, I was greatly impressed by the broad social influence that physicians seemed to wield, especially through the health commission at the area level. This suggested a widening role in area affairs, perhaps toward a mixture of health planning and community planning, a tendency for the health commission to concern itself with a broad range of matters that relate to the quality of life and to health as its measure of well-being.[21] Speaking for such a tendency was the decision in 1969 by the Santiago Region of South Oriente Province to merge other commissions with the health commission on the area and regional levels. Ostensibly, the aim of this new commission was to eliminate redundant meetings and overlapping functions, and to give attention to matters which were sometimes lost among different commissions. It was also expected that the new commission would have greater visibility and be more accessible to the people of the area.[22] I do not know the outcome of the experiment or whether it was ever adopted as a model for other areas. In the meantime, one might ask whether the larger area of cooperation leads to more or less attention to concrete matters of public health under the comprehensive goal of community welfare. Already, under the category of social services, the polyclinic seemed to lean toward an incorporation of the welfare function.[23]

With respect to the role of the physician in the area health commission, it appeared that his influence was greatest in rural areas, along with similar influence by teachers, while in urban areas, the representatives of lay organizations tended to be more assertive. The lay-professional conflict which was sometimes expressed in the health commissions was moderated by several factors, among which were the following: (1) the agenda of the commissions tended to be set by the technical representatives, (2) the sharing of common political orientations facilitated compromise, and (3) the budget tended to be generous in all areas of public health. But one well-placed foreign observer (who served as a consultant in Cuba) noted that conflict on nontechnical matters was often decided in favor of community and political representatives.[24]

From Passive to Active Mode of Health Promotion

My attention here to the sector, health commission, community health worker, and lay volunteer has been aimed at understanding the developing role of the community interface. The latter is a key element which differentiates revolutionary from prerevolutionary approaches to many health problems, especially those which call for health education, case findings, and follow-up care, not to mention the work of hygiene and sanitation. The change from a predominantly passive mode to an active mode of health protection under the revolution was simply impossible without an active neighborhood interface and lay involvement. It is reasonable, moreover, to suggest that it was the active mode which had produced the great Cuban achievements in public health during the revolutionary years.[25]

ORIGINS OF THE AREA POLYCLINIC

Having noted the position of the area polyclinic as the focus of the Cuban health system (a focus, incidentally, which increases in the next period), I will attempt to integrate previous lines of discussion by specifying the influences which shaped the area polyclinic as a distinctive Cuban institution.

The Rural Health Center

For anyone who has gained the impression that the comtemporary health system is the arbitrary creation of Czech and Soviet advisors who arrived in Cuba after 1960, it is instructive to point out that the essential ingredients of the area-polyclinic were contained in the rural health centers that were proposed *in early 1959* (and later implemented) for a Rural Health Service. The rural health center of 1959-60, with Cuban, Latin American and even North American origins, turns out to be very similar in general form and philosophical content to the polyclinic described above. Like the polyclinic, the rural health center was administratively independent of the hospital; the rural center integrated the public health responsibilities of a specific area; emphasis was given to liaison with organized popular participation in health promotion; and the people's health councils of the rural centers were clearly precursory to the area health commission. Given the context of agrarian reform, the center's functions and philosophy were merged early with the new ideologies and political structures of the revolution and, consequently, the demands of the rural center on the hospital and medical education systems carried political weight. As the practical internship of so many young physicians, the rural center cannot help but have been a substantial influence on the new personnel of the model polyclinic.

In part then, the decision to emphasize the polyclinic was simply a decision to improve and increase the number of rural health centers of the outpatient variety, linked by 1965 to a rationalized system of hospital services. Indeed, the terms had become somewhat interchangeable. Thus if one envisions, as I do, an organizational and political conflict between early 1959-61 development (small dispensaries and rural hospitals) and the 1961-63 rationalization of hospital services (provincial and regional administrations and service levels), one might argue that the emphasis on the polyclinic and the health area from 1965 to 1968 represents a victory of the first tendencies in the context of the second.

Mutualism

If the rural site of invention was the rural health center, the urban precursors of the model polyclinic were the small mutualist clinics and the dispensaries of the large, hospital-based, mutalist programs. Like the polyclinic, mutualist programs assumed comprehensive medical responsibilities, and, regardless of many inadequacies, they set an important tradition of physician employment and corporate responsibility, rather than purely individual responsibility. Unlike the polyclinic, however, mutualist clinics were removed from sanitary and preventive functions, were inadequately linked to hospital and speciality services, made ineffective use of auxiliary personnel and extravagant use of physicians, and were largely disconnected from a geographically defined base. But the rationalization of mutualism under regionalization from 1962 to 1963 transformed many mutualist clinics into a form that strikingly approximates the contemporary polyclinic.

Under regionalization, mutualist clinics eliminated redundant inpatient services. Programs were standardized. As membership was made transferable between different clinics, services were preferentially directed to specific geographical areas. Some clinics, in fact, were converted directly into MINSAP polyclinics before 1965.[26] Other mutualist clinics, like the well-known Clínica Reína in Havana, were made to serve the dual function of area polyclinic and mutualist program, offering identical services to both categories of patients.

Withering Away of Mutualism

The integration of mutualist and public services had long been urged by the irritable excess of hospital beds which continued in mutualism even as late as 1968,[27] after mutualist services had already been internally rationalized and, increasingly, either closed or changed into public facilities. Therefore, as rationalization independently occurred in mutualist and public sectors, attention was given to the historical contradiction between mutualist and public services. The resolution of the public-mutualist contradiction has derived from a two-way process of limitation of mutualist expansion and simultaneous improvement of public facilities. The completion of the polyclinic and health area represents a final stage in this process, for, by creating a public outpatient service that is similar in many respects to the evolving mutualist clinic, the raison d'être of mutualism disappears, the need of the consumer to avoid the second class care of public institutions and the high cost and insecurities of private medical care. A "withering away of mutualism" was thus expected and, as a sign of this anticipation, the budget of mutualism was included after 1967 within the budget of MINSAP. Mutualism formally ended its existence in 1970 by ending new memberships, eliminating monthly dues, and equalizing attention to members and nonmembers. The last mutualist clinic to cease independent existence was the Centro Benéfico.[28]

Casas de Socorro

The public sector, favored by the separate municipal administration of Havana, created a tradition of public services which also seems to have pointed, however modestly, in the direction of the polyclinic. As early as 1930, Havana was divided into eight districts, and each was served by an outpatient facility known as a *cuerpo de guardia* or *casa de socorro*, (roughly translated: aid station) that was staffed by physicians, dentists, and nurses. The staffing of these clinics was so highly politicized that, in the 1934 conservative counterrevolution under Mendieta-Batista, these dispensaries were occupied by police forces. Similar services existed in a few cities of the interior. Unfortunately, these services seem not to have been notably expanded in the ensuing years, and, depending on economic circumstances, patients moved away from the insufficient services of the *casas de socorro* to the outpatient services of the larger public hospitals in Havana.

The Czechoslovakian and Soviet Experiences

Much was learned from the Czech experience. The polyclinic was the outpatient category of the Czech model, and, after 1962, Cuban outpatient services of regional and provincial hospitals were often referred to as polyclinics. (But the term was used much earlier in presocialist Cuba, as in the Policlínica Nacional Cubana.) Czechoslovakia was divided into ten regions and these, in turn, into districts of between one hundred and two hundred thousand people. Here the base of hospital services was divided among pediatric, obstetrical-gynecological, and general hospitals, each with an outpatient facility which included, under direction of the same department heads, whatever specialty services were offered in the hospital. Some physicians alternated service between hospital and polyclinic, while other physicians provided home services. This structure led to a gulf between home services and the hospital-polyclinic. Meanwhile the hospitals, strongly emphasizing specialization, tended to be smaller than the optimum size and outpatient services were often overspecialized without adequate support facilities.[29] The Cubans, thus, borrowed from the Czechs precisely at a time when the key problem was recognized as the integration of general and specialty services, outpatient and inpatient services, and primary and secondary levels of care.[30] This experience was one factor in the Cuban design for primary specialization of services in the area polyclinics. In any case the Cuban system seems to have gone somewhat farther toward integration of all primary personal health services and public health functions in the polyclinic. In Czechoslovakia, the Centers of Hygiene and Epidemiology were organized separately at the level of region and district, along with separate services for women, children, and factory workers. The Czech system emphasized the integration of different categories of care, but this integration was imperfectly achieved in substantive organization.[31] The Czech system, however, was conceived in an earlier period of medical-technological progress when the costs of nonintegration were less remarkable. Thus, the Czechoslovakian experience and advancing medical technology together pointed toward the elimination of the solo office practitioner and the overspecialization of the polyclinic.

TRAINING OF PHYSICIANS

The medical school that was transformed in the first years of revolution was indeed a new school. Its newness derived primarily from new people with new values in old roles, making practical decisions in the face of great difficulties. Old roles were significantly modernized, however, in rather obvious directions: internship and residency programs, expanded teaching functions in hospitals and polyclinics, and institutionalization of new medical schools in Santiago and Santa Clara. New philosophies of health care and revolutionary camaraderie led to new styles, but few structural or curricular changes, except that epidemiology, social medicine, family health, and statistics were added as new courses, new additions to the old curriculum.

The most significant structural experimentation was the escalated vertical internship, ended in 1965, which had as its goal the rapid formation of specialists. The period, from 1962 to 1965, of crash formation of specialists reflected not only the urgency caused by medical emigration, but also the human resource needs made apparent by the rationalization of services under the Czech model and the expansion of provincial and regional service levels. Significantly, this program was terminated in 1965 when the Ministry of Public Health also turned its attentions on the health area and the "Integral Polyclinic." The purpose of medical education, as perceived in 1965, was similar to the early aims of the rural physician: to create an integral physician, one who was prepared to give primary clinical services at the polyclinic level and to integrate these functions with other tasks demanded at that level, health education and community work. Thus, it has developed that every physician is not only required to perform hospital and polyclinic services (wherever possible); he is also required to give time separately to activities in health education and community work. The rotating internship, compulsory for all students after 1965 (but compulsory for many after 1961), included, along with rotation in the various clinical departments, a rotation through the Department of Hygiene and Epidemiology of MINSAP.

The rationalization and regionalization of hospitals included, of course, all teaching facilities, the effect of which was to enhance the sense of responsibility of a health unit to a given population (as opposed to the passive attitude of the prerevolutionary hospital). The students gained opportunities to see the interrelation between hospital and community and the new role of health auxiliaries who were being trained for certain community components of service. The organization of the health area and the polyclinic increased these tendencies. Like other physicians, teachers and students were required to give services in the area polyclinics, and some polyclinics near teaching hospitals had developed specialized teaching functions. The consequence had been to give Cuban medical education a very strong community orientation. One highly respected specialist in international health services research concluded, for example, that Cuban medical education was the most community-oriented of any system known to him.[32]

Earlier, it was suggested that the large numbers of new and very different students who entered medical school in 1962 and 1963 set the mood and style of the student body for the next several years. In 1968, I found a very impressive group of students, serious and highly politicized. The fifth year class was organized into three brigades, A, B, and C, who worked and studied together, with "socialist competition" between brigades. Each year the students had spent forty-five days in agricultural labor and, as they developed clinical skills, provided medical services to agricultural workers. Next to students of political science, medical students had the highest percentage of young communists within their ranks.

New Directions

Contrary to the image of "socialist rigidity" which is held by many North Americans, the highly disciplined and politicized student body had proven to be a source of enormous creativity. In particular, this creativity was evidenced in the 1968 evaluation and far-reaching redesign of medical education, which strongly reflects student experience and active participation in curriculum review.[33] The central tendency of the 1968 reforms was elimination of excessive redundancy, a problem in medical education which was neither new nor unique to Cuba. Before 1959, each course and department functioned autonomously, without special regard for the whole; after 1959, courses and departments were supposed to develop coordinated teaching efforts, but with the extremes of personnel mobility and practical difficulties of the early period, there was little opportunity to develop a perspective of the whole process. After 1965, however, graduating students had acquired greater perspective and influence, having undergone complete professional development under the revolution. In 1965, the orientation and goals of medical education gained clarity as the health area and integral polyclinic emerged against a backdrop of a familiar and systematic organization of hospital, epidemiological, and sanitary services.

The development of social medicine (under a regime of social medicine) provides a case in point. As more teachers were themselves products of the revolutionary point of view, quite naturally they included in their courses discussions, whenever relevant, of epidemiology, rural health, and social medicine, thus creating a new kind of redundancy with the expanded courses in these areas. Therefore, in 1968, epidemiology, family health, medical psychology, rural health, tropical medicine, and social medicine were largely eliminated as separate courses, while their teaching and their perspective were expected to be integrated in virtually every course.[34] This plan was further facilitated by another teaching experiment urged by students that was designed to reduce the more traditional kinds of redundancy caused by arbitrary divisions of medical departments and courses. Much of the teaching formerly performed by academic departments (pathology, pediatrics, and so forth was replaced with courses organized by physical systems (circulatory system, nervous system, and so forth) with the cooperation of all departments, including Hygiene and Epidemiology, which has emerged as a kind of special resource for other departments.

One might suppose that experience with two kinds of internships, vertical and rotating, may have offered insight into the comparative value of narrow, intensive, and integrated training versus broad, but less intensive and less integrated training. Here again, a temporary change in direction occurred in 1968. The 1965 decision, to end the emergency escalated vertical internship program in favor of uniform rotating internships, had left the structure of specialty services somewhat truncated and concentrated in Havana. But the interim production of physicians, from 1965 to 1968, was such that the projected graduation of one thousand physicians from the "whopper" 1968-69 internship promised to considerably exceed the projected requirements of rural and area services. It was decided therefore, to move in a direction which would hasten the distribution of specialty services in the next four or five years. While roughly one half of the 1968-69 sixth year students would enter the conventional rotating internship, the other half would again be placed in vertical internships. The first group went directly to the conventional two years of rural service, while the two-year service of the second group followed assignments interpreted according to the needs and capacities of residency programs and specialty requirements. Thus, 347 specialists graduated from residency training between 1962, when the residency was formally established, and spring 1969. In 1969, there were 937 physicians engaged in residency training.[35]

Before 1968, the way was prepared for the escalated program of specialty training by the expansion of teaching functions in facilities of interior provinces. In 1968, thirty-seven hospitals had teaching areas, and seven others were known as "hospital schools."[36] Since teachers were yet insufficient in some areas, professors teaching in Havana were required to spend at least one month of every year teaching in another province. Not only did this program of professional mobility, later strongly institutionalized, help to secure teaching functions and continuing education of physicians in other areas of Cuba, it also served two other functions: professors broadened their perspectives beyond the ivory tower of the university and the metropolis, and a national medical information function was served, since many university professors provided technical input to planning task forces of the Ministry of Public Health.

AUXILIARY MEDICAL PERSONNEL

Considering that a system is composed of interrelated parts, it is not surprising that one discovers parallels between the development of auxiliary personnel and the history of other health categories. The direction set in 1968 to broaden the peak of specialized physician services coincided with the effort to consolidate the base of services, the neighborhood or sector level, with its own demands for new technical personnel. The year 1968 also saw an effort to increase geographical decentralization of the training programs for auxiliary personnel of all categories. A history of the last ten years, prepared and published by the Ministry of Public Health, divides the history of auxiliary personnel into familiar-sounding periods: 1959-63; 1963-66; 1966-67; and 1968-70.

Somewhat like the prerevolutionary specialty training of physicians, the training of nurses, technicians and auxiliaries had been largely achieved for the greater part before 1960 by nonsystematic work experience. Of six small nursing schools, three were in Havana. With the exception of one small school for medical technicians, there was no organized instruction for technicians and auxiliaries. Moreover, the services of trained nurses were concentrated in mutualist and private sectors which meant that the public sector was served for the greater part by the self-trained, practical, or "empirical" nurses, many of whom had no more than three years of primary education. Nurses who were recruited from the middle class eventually found their way to the medical services of the same class.

Systematic training and utilization of medical and paramedical specialists had long been pressured by medical technology and had developed, under the revolution, as the natural complement to regionalization. The failure or resistance of the prerevolutionary Cuban system in these areas is probably explained: (1) by the abandonment of public facilities, where one found neither the resources nor the interest to modernize personnel development, and (2) by the predominance in the private and mutualist sectors of small institutions and concentration of marginal physicians who resisted pressures for more efficient organization while they languished unhappily in an archaic system of jealously guarded specialty practices and underemployed generalists. In light of this background, the Cuban success in producing increased numbers of physicians is, in some ways, less remarkable than the preparation of nursing and paramedical personnel, most of whom graduated from entirely new programs. By 1968 there were 17,085 graduates of basic training in nursing and paramedical professions and 1,470 had completed specialty training after two years of practice.[37]

The training of nursing auxiliaries began as early as 1960, evidently as a short-run solution to rapid expansion of basic services and, I would guess, emigration of some nursing personnel. Training of specialized technicians was introduced under rationalization of services in 1962 and 1963. As these programs expanded from 1963 to 1965, the secondary specialization of nursing was inaugurated, along with courses for mobility of auxiliary nurses into higher categories. Development after 1965 followed the trend set by the orientation toward the area polyclinic and rural service. The first paramedical training had been organized near existing teaching facilities, mostly in Havana. After 1965, these training programs were extended to other provinces and integrated, for the greater part, with hospital facilities. Regional decentralization of training was motivated by the need for more effective recruitment and staffing of paramedical positions outside of Havana. At the same time, however, important new training programs for technical specialists, such as cytology technicians for new cancer screening programs, were begun on the national level in Havana. By 1968, the range of paramedical education was highly developed and increasingly decentralized throughout Cuba, bringing into perspective the goal of achieving minimal paramedical requirements in all parts of Cuba, from the dusty streets of the sector to the superspecialties of the provincial hospital.

NOTES

1. Rojas Ochoa, "La red hospitalaria," pp. 8-9.

2. Navarro, p. 413.

3. By 1969 the percentage of growth in the number of beds (1958 taken as base year) for different provinces was as follows:

Camagüey	184.2
Oriente Norte	147.9
Oriente Sur	106.3
Matanzas	83.5
Pinar del Río	75.5
Las Villas	73.1
Havana (Metro)	8.7
Havana (Interior)	7.0

(Rojas Ochoa, "La red hospitalaria," p. 8.)

4. The following figures tell the story of physical changes in hospital services, along with the assault on private and mutualist services.

Table 7.2
Changes in Hospital Services: 1959-1968

	New Facilities*		Closed Facilities**	
	number	average beds***	number	average beds***
1959	4	75	1	32
1960	3	539	8	81
1961	22	69	3	58
1962	14	140	27	75
1963	6	24	81	27
1964	7	26	16	27
1965	7	46	18	16
1966	9	150	25	53
1967	10	69	13	40
1968	12	72	26	48

*all public
**probably all private and mutualist
***That is, of the new (or closed) facilities of that year.

Meanwhile, old facilities were remodeled and expanded, and some closed facilities were remodeled. As the average size jumped, the effective increases in beds available is greater than indicated in absolute numbers, given the notoriously low occupancy rates of small hospitals. (Data adapted from Rojas Ochoa, "La red hospitalaria," pp. 19 and 31.

5. The changing patterns in outpatient visits are given as follows:

Table 7.3
Percentage of Visits by Type of Facility

	1964	1965	1966	1967	1968	1969
General Hospitals	27.8	28.3	26.1	21.3	20.4	19.0
Rural Hospitals	5.6	6.1	4.7	4.3	4.0	3.2
Sub-Total	33.4	34.4	30.8	25.6	24.4	22.2
Mutualist Clinics	26.9	25.1	22.4	17.1	10.5	6.6
Special Hospitals	2.5	2.4	2.7	2.5	2.3	1.9
Polyclinics	32.3	34.3	41.7	51.4	57.6	63.3
Rural Dispensaries	4.7	3.7	2.4	2.3	2.1	3.3
Others	—	0.1	—	1.1	2.1	2.7
Totals	99.8	100.0	100.0	100.0	99.0	100.0
Base Numbers (in thousands)	11,350	12,748	13,659	16,676	19,121	21,830

From Francisco Rojas Ochoa, "El policlínico y la asistencia a pacientes ambulatorios en Cuba," *Revista Cubana de Medicina* 10 (March-April 1971) 2: 214-15.

6. Thus, for example, U.S.A.I.D. determined in certain areas of Latin America to turn clinical facilities over to predominantly birth control or family planning functions. More recently, an acquaintance, who had consulted in South Vietnam in conjunction with A.I.D., the American Medical Association, and the Thieu government in 1968, had recommended that pediatric clinics should not be greatly expanded, inasmuch as one result would be to increase the politically unstable population of urban poor.

7. The term is borrowed from Navarro, who also describes this process in terms of planning functions.

8. Three contrasting health regions are studied by Peter Orris, "The Role of the Consumer in the Cuban Health System," unpublished masters of public health dissertation, (New Haven: Yale University, 1970). His analysis shows the interaction between the health system and other organizations, which constitute a wide choice of influential channels for consumer criticism and control to be directed at health workers and their organizations. Specific examples of regions and areas are also illustrated in Ministerio de Salud Pública, *Diez Años de Salud Pública*, pp. 61-62.

9. Navarro, pp. 423-30.

10. While the nursing profession had expanded, it had not done so at a rate which matched the expansion of physicians on the one hand or various technicians and auxiliaries on the other. This seems to have been a consequence of the easy entrance and support for physician training, attracting many who otherwise would have followed the nursing profession. Meanwhile, the plans to continue the increase in the number of physicians (to a total of 17,367 in 1980, or 1/561 inhabitants) cast doubt on the prospects for increasing the ratio of nurses to physician. In 1969, there were slightly fewer nurses than physicians. See Navarro, in this regard, and also Willy De Geyndt, "The Cuban Hospital System," *World Hospitals* 8 (1970) 3: 283.

11. Dr. Mervyn Susser and Dr. Zena Stein in Cuba during August 1972. (Dr. Stein, Seminar on Cuba, Columbia University, 1972.)

12. Rojas Ochoa, "La red hospitalaria," p. 215.

13. In this regard the CDRs are extremely important, for they educate each neighborhood in the use of various health facilities, beginning with the polyclinic, where all residents, with the aid of the CDRs, are registered.

14. See note 38, in ch. 6.

15. The goal in 1968 had been set, abstractly, at ten. The smaller number probably reflects the larger facilities among concentrated urban populations, making use of existing facilities.

16. See discussion by Carlos Font Pupo, "La salud del pueblo."

17. Orris, pp. 86-90.

18. Problems that have been suggested by a number of observers. For example, Dr. Stein, Seminar on Cuba.

19. The CDR and other organizations are discussed in some detail by Orris.

20. For example, vanguard workers are expected to take the side of patients in the event of any difficulty. Communist Party members and local CDR officials are accessible, and patients are often invited to come, bringing a friend, to certain meetings of the hospital staff. (Orris, "Consumer Participation.")

21. An example of a broad role of the polyclinic is suggested indirectly in a regional planning study, Oscar R. Mazorra and Mario Montero, "Estudio demográfico de Valle de Peru," *Economía y Desarrollo* 3 (July-August) 12: 188-212. All the data for the study were supplied by the statistical section of the area polyclinic.

22. Orris, pp. 66-67.

23. Most social security functions are now taken care of by the Ministry of Labor. The welfare function of the polyclinic needs further study and clarification. Its social work seems limited to medical problems.

24. Navarro notes that in instances of conflict, the community viewpoint, represented by the Health Commission, is often predominant.

25. This change is precisely the quality that distinguishes the work in the contemporary period from all preceding work, dating from the public health efforts of Romay. It has been the essential ingredient to achieve the control of such long elusive health problems as tuberculosis, leprosy, and malaria, not to mention the better known examples of immunization. The mass organizations make it possible, for example, to reach specific populations, such as women in ages recommended for early detection of cancer. To see how this is true in the case of leprosy, see Miguel A. González Prendes "Informe del relator general" (National Conference on Norms of Leprosy Control, 1962) *Revista Cubana de Medicina* 1 (November-December) 6: 45-50. The success of this program is suggested by the decrease of hospitalization for leprosy patients. See Rojas Ochoa, "La red hospitalaria," p. 16.

26. As was the private psychiatric hospital, Pérez Vento, which became the Integral Polyclinic of Guanabacoa. See López Valdés, p. 69.

27. With an occupancy rate of 60%, I was told in 1968. Rojas Ochoa's statistics are similar.

28. "Esto nos permitirá iniciar la década del 70 con este tipo de institución eradicada." See Rojas Ochoa, "La red hospitalaria," p. 4. Marking the end of an era, one might wish to contemplate the role of such an old institution in Cuba. All its defects aside, it would be important to remember it as a source of experimentation and innovation both before and after 1959. In 1965-66, for example, mutualist clinics experimented and reported on the sleep-in parent as a nurse's assistant in pediatric hospitalization, an innovation which has since been promulgated as a norm of hospital practice. See Antonio González Romero and René Hernández Viñas, "La madre como acompañante del niño hospitalizado en nuestras unidades," *Revista Cubana de Pediatría* 38 (August 1966) 4: 475-84. Other advanced mutualist hospitals were outstanding in internal education and review of medical work. The eclectic orientation of Cuban medicine seems, however, to ensure continued innovations, with many foreign scholarships, visiting professors, collective administration and consumer participation.

29. See Weinerman, pp. 78-87.

30. See Dr. Stitch, p. 354.

31. Personal interview, Havana. 1968.

32. Navarro, p. 418.

33. This finding, supported by the work of Vicente Navarro and my own research, contrasts sharply with Hugh Thomas' conclusion that "though students nominally participate in the running of the institutions in which they work, these are in all important respects tied to the needs of the economy, not the desires of the student." (Thomas, p. 1428.) The work of Hochschild provides a more generous, broader, and, I think, more accurate view of the university and its students.

34. This is described by Navarro, pp. 417-18.

35. Ministerio de Salud Pública, *Diez Años de Salud Pública*, p. 169.

36. Probably the central "university hospitals." See Ministerio de Salud Pública, *Salud Pública en Cifras, 1968*, (Havana: Ministerio de Salud Pública, 1968), table 69.

37. Ministerio de Salud Pública, *Diez Años de Salud Pública*, pp. 170-78.

8
Medicine in the Community

OUTCOME OF CONSOLIDATION

The word consolidation, which I have applied to the years 1965 through 1971, suggests unification of action, definition, and purpose — an improved consideration of a whole in contrast to its parts. But consolidation also suggests centralization, uniformity, rigidity — the domination of parts by the whole. Observers of the Cuban health endeavor were bound, therefore, to ask whether consolidation would be followed by yet another slide into bureaucratic entrenchment, a lapse in the history of creative resolution of contradictions, a stagnation in the debate over problems, solutions, and long-range goals.

Such questions are inevitably raised in the context of others: does consolidation under socialism lay the basis for future transformation, as the communist perspective demands? Or does consolidation lead to a gray mass of unresponsive bureaucracies, as the capitalist vision of socialism proclaims? But both questions are misleading insofar as they seek a definitive response. An *assumption* that socialism moves forward distracts attention from the more important question of *how* socialism moves forward, while the contrary assumption hides the magnitude of changes already introduced. And both questions mask the essential ambiguity and conflict inherent to social reality.

I therefore seek, as I have in preceding periods, to identify *predominant* rather than exclusive tendencies. With this proviso, I have concluded that the period of consolidation has not been followed by a slide into entrenchment, but rather by a period of new transformations. To see how this has been the case requires a review of the components of consolidation and of the evolving elements of its ambiguity and internal conflict. It is also necessary to outline the societal changes which compose the continuing Cuban Revolution. The elements thus identified may then be observed in concrete events of contemporary transformation in Cuban health care.

The consolidation by 1970 of the Cuban health system could be summarized in the virtual extinction of medical practice outside the authority of the Ministry of Public Health, the ending of private practice, the termination of mutualism. Comprehensive planning was effected in yearly and multiyearly planning cycles. Institutes of research, postgraduate education, programs of nonuniversity training, and all of traditional public health and sanitation were directed and planned with the ministry. A comprehensive model guided the organization of health services everywhere; the ambiguity and multiplicity of entry to the medical services system was significantly ended by the focus on the area polyclinic as the focal unit of the system.[1]

Other system characteristics, however, presented themselves as potential tensions or antagonisms for change:

1. in administration and planning, a continuing interaction between the national centralization of normative responsibilities and the decentralized concentration of administrative, operative responsibilities in the provinces, regions and areas;
2. in medical services, a tension between the centralizing tendencies of inpatient services and the decentralizing direction of outpatient services;
3. in the area polyclinic, a tension between its relation to the community and its relation to the hospital system;
4. in medical education, a tension between the community service philosophy of medical care and the dominant role of hospital-based learning experiences and specialty training;
5. in the community of medical workers, a difference in perspective between physicians and nonphysicians; and
6. in the evaluation of health work, the continuing experience of service deficiencies and consumer complaints, notwithstanding the many well-intentioned efforts at resolving them.

Features which could be hypothesized to influence the form of problem resolution included the structured representation of lay community organizations in health activities, politically-supported mechanisms for hearing consumer complaints, and the evolving socialist character of the larger society.

CONTINUING SOCIALIST REVOLUTION

The year 1970 marked the close of a period, begun in 1968, that was known as the "revolutionary offensive." The objective of the offensive, to use the combative terms which had come to express the Cuban situation, was to mobilize the resources of the country in order to achieve a dramatic new level of economic and social development, a superior base for the construction of communist society. The plan represented at once the evolving goals of the revolution and a critical evaluation of the strengths, weaknesses, and problems of the eclectic first years.

The early years had proven effective in mobilizing citizens for the tasks of defense, rural development, hurricane disaster relief, public health programs, and the famous literacy campaign. As land reform, industrialization, and agricultural diversification efforts disrupted the previous organization of sugar production, mobilization of urban labor — much of it from service and bureaucratic occupations — became a useful means of meeting labor requirements of the harvest. This measure was also intended to serve the ideological objective of integrating manual and intellectual labor. Meanwhile, the initial goals of full employment, rural development, and increased real income for working people — especially for the prerevolutionary poor — led to a shift under the crush of scarcity conditions to a regulated consumer economy which guaranteed equal distribution of goods and services by rationing consumer items and decreasing salary stratification. Cuba's inability to produce or import other than strictly essential consumer goods in the barest amounts, after an unwillingness to compromise the initial goals of economic investment and income transfer, argued in favor of an economic strategy to abandon most free market pricing systems and to utilize methods of mobilization and moral incentives to secure effective labor utilization. The program of moral incentives was additionally intended to produce positive changes in social values and to elevate the meaning of work.[2]

Elsewhere within the economic sphere, the first years after 1959 had revealed the pitfalls, if not the outright impossibility, of attempting to swiftly implement the watchwords of agricultural diversification and domestic industrialization in a neocolonial single cash crop island society which was faced with an American blockade and covert economic sabotage. Without abandoning available international capitalist market relations, the Cuban economy had to secure a position within the socialist world community. In particular, it was realized that industrialization had to adjust itself to agricultural goals and that agricultural planning had to begin with the stabilization and technical perfection of sugar production rather than its abandonment. Initial planning estimated the optimum level of annual sugar production to be some ten million tons, a target which was set overoptimistically for 1970, the conclusion of the revolutionary offensive. The year 1970, then, was a difficult one not only because it ended three years of sacrifice but because in important respects the revolutionary offensive was unsuccessful.

The offensive ended with the conclusion of the sugar harvest in late spring of that year, and the remaining months (and indeed the following years) were marked by retrospective analysis, criticism, and self-criticism at all levels and regions of Cuban society. Cuba had *not* failed to mobilize resources, human or material, and workers had not failed to respond to moral incentives.[3] The scale of mobilization was simply beyond the capacity of the administrative and political structures of the society. Production techniques and level of mechanization were unequal to the 1970 target, and the negative effects of minor technical difficulties were multiplied in an effort to meet that target. As a result of this stress, other economic sectors were disrupted and set back. Faced with this experience in 1970, Cuba, now highly socialized after ten years of revolution (the last small business had been closed to preempt black marketeering), was turned toward new courses[4]. On the one hand, she sought strategies that would more securely guarantee economic stability and labor productivity and would ease the sacrifices demanded of the Cuban people. On the other hand, she sought to gradually move away from reliance on large campaigns of voluntary mass mobilization and toward political reform that would broaden democratic participation and improve decentralized administration. Political democratization and decentralization were not only worthy ends in themselves; they were recognized as essential for the optimum functioning of the economy.

The early and rapid nationalization of the economy had placed immense responsibilities in what was essentially a *provisional* government. Notwithstanding efforts at regionalism, particularly in planning, the overall pattern of social administration was set by the many sectoral hierarchies (construction, sugar industry, light industry, labor, health, and so forth) that led to the Council of Ministers in Havana. The redistribution of this wealth of administrative responsibility was the task that was now thrust on the agenda, and at the same time, the task of transition from a provisional revolutionary government to the formation of a new socialist state.[5]

Before examining this transformation, it is worth adding that mobilization and other characteristics of the period before 1970 had other consequences which were not always summarized in the analysis of production figures. One indicator that racial and sexual inequalities were decreasing was that counterrevolutionaries and *disgustados* (those who are displeased with the revolution but do not act against it), increasingly complained that Blacks were getting everything, morals were declining, and women were losing the "enchantment of femininity." Income levelling, equalization of opportunity, and active recruitment of women into the labor force began to undermine the infrastructures of racism and sexism.[6]

Mobilization in the first ten years also contributed to a heightened social conscience and understanding. Public visibility and popular participation in the process of developing, implementing, and criticizing major social policies led large numbers of ordinary people to acquire an understanding of socioeconomic matters that is unknown in many societies.

The Matanzas Experiment

In forging a path through debate and criticism toward the new socialist state, it was decided to experimentally implement some of the reform proposals in one of the Cuban provinces. The evaluation of this experience would then provide a practical basis for the specification of new forms in a socialist constitution. Proposals were thus put to the test in Matanzas province from 1973 to 1975. Matanzas, it is said, was chosen for its outstanding record for meeting production targets after 1969. (Before that, the Mantanzas record was poor, marred by counterrevolution and weak party structure.)

It is probably more than coincidental for the theme of this book that the person who undertook to lead and build the party in Matanzas was previously the minister of public health, from 1960 to 1969. A Rebel Army physician, Dr. Ramón Machado Ventura, was anxious to try his hand in political work that was closer to the process of production than public health. Today he serves as a member of the influential Political Bureau of the Central Committee of the Communist Party.

Two key ingredients of the Matanzas experiment were the creation of popular assemblies and the separation of party and government functions. Elected assemblies (*asambleas de poder popular*) were created at municipal, regional, and provincial levels. At the municipal level, delegates were elected by universal suffrage and secret ballot, from open nominations in each precinct of the municipality. This assembly of precinct delegates held monthly meetings and elected an executive council. The municipal assembly named delegates to the regional assembly, while the regional assemblies in their turn elected the delegates to the provincial assembly. A system of accountability was imposed, and each municipal delegate, for instance, was required to give an accounting (*rendición de cuentas*) at a public precinct meeting held every three months. I had opportunity to attend two such meetings in the city of Matanzas in March 1976. The occasions were taken very seriously, with the delegates giving account of innumerable municipal actions, particularly those that had been questioned in the previous period by precinct residents. The accounting was sometimes rejected, even strongly, by the gathered citizens. In one precinct, the delegate was, I think, a mechanic; in the other the delegate happened to be a polyclinic director. Less than one-fourth of the municipal delegates were women, a statistic which was loudly bemoaned by the party after the first municipal elections in 1975.

Party members, as I have previously commented, had by 1968 come to play a loose role as orienters, cadre builders, and general troubleshooters. Over time, the role of the party was often confused with the role of government. In the years of mobilization, multiple lines of authority, and ingenious working out of channels, party members not only examined problems but implemented solutions, even by intervention. One consequence was to produce an excessively diffused accountability and, in particular, *unaccountability* among administrative functionaries who looked to the party rather than to the people. Hardly need I add that superhuman expectations were often cast for party members. A phenomenon which in earlier years was correctly associated with flexibility and innovation was increasingly an obstacle. In Matanzas, then, the party helped in orienting the new political experiment, but scrupulously respected the lines of accountability created under the new assemblies.

The Socialist Constitution

The Socialist Constitution which was adopted by universal plebiscite in Fall 1975 reformulated the successful features of the Matanzas experiment for general application in the nation. Under the guidance of the party, which held its first national congress in December 1975, the system of peoples' assemblies was extended throughout Cuba in 1976. The mechanism of the regional assembly was eliminated, however, as excessively hierarchic; but the number of Cuban provinces was increased from six to thirteen to give adequate expression to functional regionalism. The new constitution affirms the rights and duties of the Cuban citizen and the irrevocable nature of the socialist transformation. Protection of health is one of the rights declared by the document. The constitution also reaffirms the Cuban Family Code, a notable document of social principles and feminist reform, which was already adopted in 1974 after a year of heated public discussion.

In another, related, institutional development, change is occurring in the role of labor unions. In keeping with the drive for greater administrative accountability, it appears appropriate that unions should be less involved with enterprise management (as was the tendency under mobilization) than with the presentation and defense of the immediate interests of workers. Technical expertise for management is now prized equally with, if not more than, ideological criteria. Indeed, accumulated experience has modified the extremes of opposing political economic viewpoints, and many who had early fallen into disgrace around technical issues have regained a measure of respectability.[7]

Economic trends include: increasing sophistication in economic planning, membership in the Soviet-Eastern Europe trade community, utilization of flexible price mechanisms for nonessential consumer goods, improvement of transportation, increasing mechanization in agriculture, revision and decreased reliance on mobilization techniques and moral incentives, and greater encouragement of production by means of an emphasis on administrative responsibility and moderate material incentives. But mobilization and moral appeal continue to be central in the Cuban economic and ideological perspective and were much more visible in March 1976 than I had anticipated. The change is one of scale and relative emphasis. Mobilization now tends to be directed to tasks that are closer to the immediately experienced self-interests of workers; the best examples are provided by the mini-brigades which build housing destined for poorly housed coworkers. During my last visit, the national office of the Ministry of Public Health was employing volunteers to renovate an old hospital, adapting it to serve as the headquarters of a new Institute of Health Development. Signs in a radio workers' cafeteria (there are free lunches in schools and industry) announced voluntary labor mobilizations to paint houses or harvest potatoes; on one early Sunday morning, I joined public health workers to assist, as in the past, in harvesting sugar cane.

The prices of rationed items, which still include many necessities, continue to be deflated to assure universal availability, while the prices of free market items (an increasing category) vary greatly and can be quite high. But in contrast to 1968, there were in 1976 hardly any lines at the shops and few interruptions in the supply of essentials. Also contrasting with 1968 are the increasing number and attendant problems of automobiles, most of which are destined for use by state enterprises and some, under specified criteria, for individual use. A superhighway joins Cienfuegos and Havana, and track is being laid for a modern railway that will run the length of the island.

But to those who visit Havana, the most visible change since 1968 is that, for the first time within the revolutionary years, buildings of all kinds are being painted and renovated. This change does not indicate the end of efforts to restrict the growth of Havana (considered overgrown in the presocialist era), but rather the beginning of a period which will also provide some of the less essential amenities of life. Clubs, small restaurants, and entertainment are highly visible and patronized, even though in the case of clubs and fine restaurants the prices seem somewhat high. The prices, however, do not appear to affect the confluence of complexions, dress, and manners. Domestic recreation facilities are being constructed along with tourist accommodations for the increasing flow of visitors from abroad, particularly from Canada and the Caribbean. Tourism, of course, is only one expression of the near collapse of the United States sponsored blockade of Cuba.

Cubans speak proudly of their impressive system of schools, especially the expanding program of boarding schools in the countryside where secondary students combine study with manual work and outdoor sports. (Each school, incidentally, employs a full-time nurse and one pediatrician is designated for every five schools. Health education is emphasized, and a large number of students participate in Red Cross brigades, performing first aid and sanitary functions.) The quality of life is also measurably improved by standardized legal and judicial processes. Here the role of community-based popular tribunals continue to be important, but proceduralization also formulates functions for the previously disparaged law profession.

The happy irony for Cuba today is that the present period of great institutional change also conveys a sense of stability and general security. Given the economic and political vitality and the visible improvement in the living conditions of the vast majority of the population, there is a feeling in the country that Cuban socialism is coming of age.

CRITIQUE OF HEALTH ORGANIZATION

The post-1970 changes just described are rooted in the constructive critique of 1970 conditions; this is also true of the health system. However, in the case of the health system, the changes that are occurring are more surprising to the outside observer because the system appeared successfully consolidated, although not without problems, in 1968-1972. This appearance was supported by epidemiological data indicating a marked improvement in the health status of the population by 1970.[8] Certainly the pre-1970 developments were sufficient to impress many foreign visitors, including myself. Although I had no data, other than unstructured direct observations and the reported observations of others, a significant level of consumer satisfaction seemed to prevail. The community focus of medical training and service was, I concluded, highly developed.

But I was intrigued to ask, at the conclusion of my early analysis, what would be the future of neighborhood regionalization, whose development was only beginning in 1968 and at that time was regarded as a "final stage" of structural development? Was it here, perhaps, that new roles could develop which would serve to reduce some of the problems of impersonality and discontinuity of services that were visible in the area polyclinic and the hospital? Secondly, I asked, given the dominant career model of technical specialization, how would the socialist goal of leveling within the ranks of health workers be pursued? How would the community focus of primary care workers compete with the somewhat distant community focus of the (apparently) higher-ranking specialties? To what extent could leveling continue to be served by rationalized salary structures and "going where the revolution called"? To these questions, I added another: considering, in particular, the dominant role of physicians in the formulation of health policy, how could the technical development of services be *limited* or restrained in accord with resource limitations and overall social goals, and not merely rationalized and systemized? Other observers raised related questions. Would the area polyclinic continue to develop as a relatively automonous organization in the health system? *Should* it continue to enjoy such a degree of independence from the hospital? Perhaps it would be better and more efficient to integrate the area polyclinic under the hospital system?

All of these questions were debated by Cubans; indeed, many of the tendencies observed in 1970-1972 appear shaped by them — the requirement of voluntary labor by medical students, the new teaching activities in polyclinics, the expansion of the role of medical psychology and sociology, the development of family-oriented care, the exalted position of epidemiological and administrative specialties, the increasing decentralization of training and services, and, as we have seen, an emphasis on experimentation.

The Plaza Experiment

One very important experiment, begun in 1972, was conducted in the new "Plaza Polyclinic," named after the central Havana district and housing project adjacent to the Plaza of the Revolution. Designed to serve an expanding population of prerevolutionary poor who were now occupying new housing in the area, the polyclinic was also intended as a teaching center which could serve as a model of health care with a community bent. It was here that many of the features and roles of the contemporary model were first introduced.

The formulation of models for this experiment was based on accumulated critiques of existing services. The models partly evolved from the apparent difficulties in providing students with genuine community experience in existing institutions. If students could not gain intensive community contact under the prevailing models, how could it be imagined that practicing health workers were in contact with the community?

Another explanation for the Plaza experiment rests on the *newness* of the facility and the expanding number of residents of the area who had not yet begun to orient their health care needs toward the polyclinic. Given the prerevolutionary concentration of medical resources in Havana, teaching activities were previously located in established institutions, already passively receiving an abundance of patients. In the case of Plaza Polyclinic, then, there was a greater need — as had been the case with the rural health centers — to develop an *active* mode of care. Not surprisingly, the second polyclinic to implement the new models of service and teaching was

"Alamar," another new polyclinic in a town development of the same name, ten miles east of Havana near Guanabacoa. As in any new facility, an opportunity existed to model the organization according to emerging theory, relatively unfettered by previous patterns.

The experience of the Plaza experiment along with other studies of the health system,[9] pointed not only to new patterns for medical training, but also to new models of work in the polyclinic, new models of relations with the community, and an implicit criticism of the prevailing patterns of health care.

Assessment Commission for Medicine in the Community

In 1974, the Ministry of Public Health designated an interdisciplinary commission to "elaborate the conceptualization of community medicine within the Marxist-Leninist and socialist ideology and character of the health system."[10] The precise motivations for establishing this commission are unclear to me, but it was part of an effort to make sense out of contrary tendencies within the health system, bringing health activities under sharper ideological analysis, a tendency that was consistent with the prevailing thrust in Cuba toward greater institutional accountability and labor discipline. The commission also seems to have figured as part of Cuban preparations for participation in the Interamerican Conference on Community Medicine set for 1975 in Costa Rica. Logically, the commission included leaders of the Plaza experiment.

The Assessment Commission for Medicine in the Community began its work by first considering the different meanings of community medicine under capitalism and socialism. In capitalist societies, they concluded, the word community serves to obfuscate class contradictions; for in most instances the so-called community medicine programs are in fact special programs for the poor. By contrast, under socialism a community of interests prevails; the exploitation of man by man based on class has been eradicated. As health care is made accessible to all, shifting from private to socialist, elitist to popular, and mercantile to humanist, community medicine is created. The community aspect of medicine, then, is primarily a consequence of socialism. But while the need to invent a separate community medicine disappears, another question, both technical and political, gains primacy: how is medicine to be integrated into the community? This question, conceived also as task, theory, and practice, is what the commission then considered to be its area of concern — medicine in the community.

The commission vigorously pursued its evaluation and issued its assessment and recommendations. Coming from another quarter, the assessment might easily have been interpreted as an exaggerated attack on Cuban medicine. Reviewing user complaints, the commission noted: "insufficient appointments; inadequate facilities; physicians frequently in bad humor, hurried and multi-referring; cancellation or substitution of consultations .. .; waiting lists; and pilgrimage through different hospitals in search of technological support (complementary tests)."[11] A "tremendous" pressure was felt by the regional and provincial hospitals and institutes, and, the same report continued, "Particularly worrisome is the overload to which emergency services are subjected, overutilized to treat problems which are not in themselves urgent."

But how could such a situation exist in a country that had focused its attention on the area polyclinic? Precisely, the Commission on Medicine in the Community answered, because the conceptual focus of the system was not adequately matched by substantive focus. There was, in the words of the commission, "a non-correspondence between the conceptual and the structural framework of the polyclinic" that was evidenced in the polyclinic's relative poverty of human and material resources. Idealistic staffing methods (in particular the exchange of personnel between hospital and polyclinic, which in theory gave primacy to the community focus) made it difficult for a patient to always or even frequently be seen by the same person. The opposite was true as well. Physicians had trouble following a single patient through the various stages of treatment. Due to the movement of personnel and a somewhat diffuse concept of teamwork, exactly who had responsibility for a given patient at a given time was sometimes unclear and easily overlooked. The tug-of-war between hospital and polyclinic had not gone easily for the latter, and meanwhile the patient, in the middle, was suffering.

Polyclinics, which tended to lack full-time staffs, did not have polyclinic physicians but rather had so many "physician hours." Performing polyclinic duties only one or two days a week, physicians easily overrelied on referrals. Understandably, teaching physicians, who worked under the same conditions, were also pressured to work in the same fashion, removed from the community and its problems. Although the political interests of students were often successfully directed toward the community, this interest was soon frustrated by the noncorrespondence between concept and structure. Technical training and interests continued to be hospital bound — even when they were developed in the polyclinic. Insufficient training to understand the concerted activities of community health promotion contributed to a technical disinterest in primary care, and the hospital's dominance of training continued the tendency to underrate the social, psychological, and ecological aspects of health. The orientation toward prevention was similarly weakened, favoring in practice, if not in theory, the cure of disease over the promotion of health. The physician was in the polyclinic, but his mind was in the hospital.

The mediocre physician participation in the active in-the-community dimension of the area polyclinic rendered the physician essentially *passive*. The commission criticized this attribute in the strongest terms: "Although the purpose of our health system is to dispense increasing satisfaction of health needs of our people, the physician who is formed in the molds inherited from the past does not tend to practice this service-oriented medicine. Instead of serving, the physician tends to be served by the community and its people, in conformity with a medicine of consumption."[12]

Leaving none of the exalted concepts of Cuban socialist health organization untouched, the commission also castigated the polyclinic for deficient teamwork and the health system in general for incomplete lay participation. The polyclinic director was the only person who could be counted on with any certainty to have a view of the whole task of the health area, and this limited distribution of organizational consciousness served along with other factors to stifle teamwork.[13] At the primary level of attention, there were thus few real health teams, and the feeble teamwork which existed had insufficient tie with the community, where the leadership capacity of lay volunteers remained underdeveloped. The latter shortcoming was declared unacceptable, not only in light of the objective of community-medical integration, but also unacceptable from the view of the dominant ideology of Cuban socialism: "In our country mobilization of the people is significant in its own right, for it makes possible the construction of socialism and foments, with this social practice, the development toward a new revolutionary consciousness — communist consciousness."[14] The community, declared the commission, should pass from object to subject of health programs, participating in planning, execution, and control; the health team should adopt an advisory role, sharing its technical understanding and letting itself be transformed by this practice.

In order to avoid undue emphasis on the problems of the polyclinic as the source of agitation for reform, it should be recalled that problems of discontinuity in hospital care were also considered and also pointed toward reform. For example, an analysis in 1970 of pediatric hospital readmissions led to a program of discharging high-risk children not to their parents but first to the area health facility, designating a specific health worker personally responsible for the subsequent recuperation of the child. It was not merely the polyclinic, but also the hospital which stood to gain from an improvement of medicine in the community. But the thrust for new development, nonetheless, came primarily from the polyclinic, or perhaps one should say from the tension between the hospital and polyclinic. In this sense, the outcome of the work of the Advisory Commission on Medicine in the Community could be considered the ideology of a "polyclinic movement" which sought hegemony over the entire health system.

A NEW MODEL FOR THE AREA POLYCLINIC

The changes proposed by the Advisory Commission and further refined in the planning process of the Ministry of Public Health were expressed in a new model of work for the area polyclinic. Many of its features were already present in the Plaza experiment and were soon applied in 1974-1975 in Alamar. By March 1976, there were five model polyclinics in Cuba and twenty were targeted for 1980. Meanwhile, all area polyclinics were mandated to develop plans to incorporate elements of the new model in accord with local conditions. This long-run transformation of Cuba's polyclinics is being expedited, no doubt, by the tendency to use the new polyclinics as teaching settings.

Sectorization of Full-time Polyclinic Work

The new polyclinic differs from the previous model chiefly by its method of work. The polyclinic's responsibility for the health of the people in its area is entrusted to physician-nurse teams and the work of these teams is "sectorized" in the fashion of a geographically-bound capitation system. That is, just like the community work of the sanitarian, whose work was already sectorized in the 1968 model, the work of each team is directed exclusively toward a specified geographical segment of the polyclinic's area. A pediatrician-nurse team, for example, is thus responsible for the health promotion of all children in a specified area.

Two kinds of activities replace the former requirement of hospital work. On the one hand, the physician-nurse teams are expected to spend a relatively large amount of time (about twelve hours per week) making home visits, or in related community work such as health education or liaison with community groups. On the other hand, the physician dedicates time to "intra-consultation." That is, instead of referring patients away to specialists, the primary care physician participates directly as a third party in consultations between patient and specialists. Although the patient may consequently follow a course of treatment with the specialist or in the hospital, the primary team follows the case and continues to schedule appropriate intra-consultations. But following the case does not include, except in special circumstances, the direct participation in hospital care by polyclinic staff physicians.

Active Medicine

A number of consequences follow from the new approach to care. The patient no longer has to wait for a centralized clinic record room to draw his chart. Instead, she or he goes directly to the team office where all records of the catchment area are located. Although the internist, for example, may not be specifically trained in family medicine, the new organization of health care delivery is expected to promote a family and social approach, since the internist (who makes home visits) will deal with all the adult members in a dwelling and neighborhood. Health activities of lay organizations are also expected to be improved by the direct involvement of physicians and nurses. The staff of the polyclinic holds regular meetings with the citizens of each sector in order to ensure continuing community participation in the protection and promotion of health. Finally, an important consequence of the clinical team's having a specified case load is that preferential, systematic, and aggressive attention is given to persons of high risk. On a visit to a primary health team, one therefore sees not only the actual patient charts, but also the card files of patients with appropriate flags indicating risk categories. For each category, the team follows a specific protocol of case review. Thus the obstetrics-gynecology team will routinely request to see the mother of a high birthweight newborn to be certain that the mother is not diabetic. And hypertensive adult will be regularly examined by the adult medicine team (internist-nurse).

Table 8.1*
Detection of Hypertension, Alamar, January-June 1975

Sectors	Universe	Population (No.)	Examined (%)	Hypertensives Detected	Rate per 1000 Adults
A-1	1,300	657	50.5	71	10.3
A-2	1,388	600	43.2	71	11.8
B	2,359	995	42.2	85	8.5
C	1,691	995	58.8	92	9.2
D	1,843	752	40.8	34	4.5
Community	8,581	3,999	46.6	353	8.8

*Source: José A. Fernández Sacasas, et al., "Programa integral de salud para el adulto según el modelo de medicina en la comunidad," *Revista Cubana de Administración de Salud*, 1 (July-December 1975) 3-4, p. 163.

The polyclinic physician, then, is responsible not only for the patients who appear in the polyclinic but also for those who do not. The methodology for aggressively serving the community according to a prioritization by risk is called, after the Soviet fashion, *dispensarización*, but could be simply called, I think, *active medicine*. In the first six months of the Alamar experiment in 1975, targets for adult medicine included: adolescents, the aged, heart disease, hypertension, diabetes, stroke, asthma, tuberculosis, and citological exams for cervical and uterine cancer. Table 8.1 presents the adult population served by the polyclinic and the number examined by adult medicine teams, broken down by sectors and showing the numbers of hypertensive patients detected. Given the number of cases detected, the polyclinic administration then reviewed the fulfillment of patient follow-up goals. This experience is presented in Table 8.2. The role of home visits for this category of patients is suggested by the low completion of scheduled return visits to the polyclinic (32.4%) compared to the overcompletion of plans for home visits (127%).

Table 8.2*
Follow-up for Hypertension, Alamar, January-June 1975

Sector	Cases Detected	Office Consultations Planned	Realized	(%)	Home Visits Planned	Realized	(%)
A-1	71	142	43	(30)	36	65	(181)
A-2	71	142	66	(47)	36	66	(183)
B	85	170	41	(24)	43	42	(98)
C	92	184	26	(14)	46	24	(52)
D	34	68	53	(78)	17	29	(170)
Community	353	706	229	(32)	178	226	(127)

*Source: José Fernández Sacasas, et al., "Programa integral de salud para el adulto según el modelo de medicina en la comunidad," *Revista Cubana de Administración de Salud*, 1 (July-December 1975) 3-4, p. 164.

Teamwork

Teamwork, which was regarded as deficient in the critique of the "old" polyclinic, is subject to increasingly sophisticated analysis. In part, this is owed to psychologists and sociologists who are beginning to make contributions in health matters, particularly *via* the role of the medical psychologist in the model polyclinic. To the critique of the old area polyclinic, the social-psychological perspective added the concepts of atomization and alienation of the patient, closed professional hierarchies, and narrow technical perspectives: the contradiction between the presumed psychological strength of a doctor-patient relationship under a solo-practitioner model and the critized alienation of the doctor-patient relationship under the polyclinic model. Under the former model, the patient may have felt better even when he did not get better. Perhaps the structure of the polyclinic, with its complex organization to integrate multiple levels of technical sophistication, should be scrapped? To this question, which was more than rhetorical, a medical psychologist replied as follows.

Notwithstanding [the criticisms of the polyclinic], we believe that the structure should not be modified *a priori*, for the failure is not to be found in the structure, but in the lack — at the base of the structure — of primary horizontal teams which may facilitate communication and integration of health activities. It is these teams, and the changes in the concepts of medical practice, that will be called in the future to modify or maintain the essence of the present structure of the polyclinics.[15]

The primary horizontal teams, then, form the nucleus of the model polyclinic. In addition to having the usual characteristics of teamwork (practical understanding of interrelated, well-defined roles in the light of common objectives), these teams are expected to accept new members from time to time, according to specific task requirements and even to let the lines of authority within the team shift according to the same requirements. In practice, the primary horizontal teams principally consist of physicians (internist, pediatrician, or obstetro-gynecologist) and corresponding nursing staff. At the same time, these personnel are part of secondary horizontal teams, defined by overlapping work in a particular sector. For example, an internist-nurse team may work exclusively in one sector, but there may be only one obstetro-gynecologist team and only one pediatrician team to serve two sectors. (See Diagram 8.1.) Thus, the secondary team of each internist-nurse includes a pediatrician-nurse and an obstetro-gynecologist nurse; the secondary horizontal team of the pediatrician-nurse includes two internists-nurses and one obstetro-gynecologist nurse; and likewise for the obstetro-gynecologist nurse. Finally, the complete sector team also includes a sanitarian, perhaps a field nurse, and lay health activists.

Diagram 8.1
Primary and Secondary Horizontal Medical Teams in Two Sectors

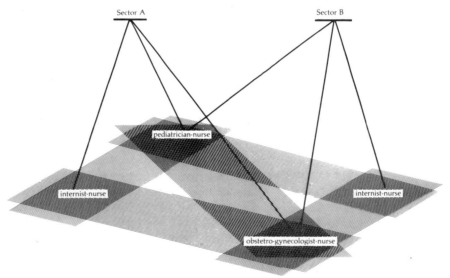

The primary horizontal team, to be able to effect changes in the environment, temporarily includes a member from the environmental team. In other situations, a social worker, psychologist, or a hospital-based specialist. But the same may be said of still other situations which call for lay participation (immunization, follow-up, health education). In such conditions, the team is expected to flexibly modify the lines of its authority, even of its leadership, to meet the task at hand.

Departing from the nucleus of primary and secondary horizontal teams, the structure of the new polyclinic resembles the old. The polyclinic as a whole comprises the "basic team" and is guided by a director, an administrative council, and the service assembly. The latter is the institution, common to all enterprise management in Cuba, of regular assemblies of the entire work-force. The administrative council includes the leaders of secondary vertical teams: clinical, laboratory, and environmental health and epidemiology, along with labor union representation. "Primary vertical teams" include social work, psychology, estomatology (dentistry), pediatrics, maintenance, statistics, and so on.

This account of sectorization, active medicine, and teamwork, even if somewhat idealized or conceptual, completes the discussion of the model polyclinic and the core ingredients of medicine in the community. To describe it in more detail would unduly concretize a concept which is in process of substantive development. The general description provided here fits rather well the three model polyclinics which I visited in 1976 — Plaza de la Revolución, Alamar, and Reynol García in the city of Matanzas. Reviewing what I have written, I should add, however, that the focus on new characteristics and criticism of the old has diverted attention from established and successful aspects which are more prominent and visible than might be interpreted here.

Implications

The new model for the polyclinic has a number of implications which may not be obvious. First of all, it requires the training of even more physicians than the number implied by the previous model. By creating a clear vocational role for a physician exclusively dedicated to primary service in the community, the new model resolves an ambiguity which was always expressed in previous years, between the goal of training the integral physician and achieving coverage by hospital-based specialists, between the goal of community service and the goal of integration between service levels. The previous strategy of vertical integration (via academic specialties and program categories) has been modified by the prioritized strategy of horizontal integration at the base. The replacement of hospital-polyclinic rotation by the mechanism of intra-consultation, together with the definition of horizontal teamwork, creates conditions for a new set of community-bound affective relationships for the integral physician. The same process favors the advancement and integrated roles of other health workers, whose numbers and scope of training and responsibility was greatly enlarged by 1972, prior to the implementation of the new model of work. Although hardly for the first time, physician dominance is being concretely if not loudly challenged, modified by a criterion of teamwork which specifies situations where the physician is to yield team leadership to nonphysicians.

To a degree that cannot yet be specified, the turn toward medicine in the community seems to break a trend which maintained and even increased (by improving) the influence and prestige of clinical specialization. The clinical specialists, powerful on the technical committees of the ministry exerted a dominant budgetary claim, even when the social medical perspectives determined the overall philosophy and structure. The trend in the flow of resources to the parts of the structure seemed to favor the former, and with the always expansive appetite of hospital and specialist technology for greater shares of public funds, it seems inevitable that the polyclinic perspective would be constantly threatened, particularly if it did not assert and expand its role and particularly after the budgetary generosity of the sixties was tempered by the pragmatism of the seventies. Meanwhile, only an effective organization of primary services could protect the hospital system for its uniquely specialized contribution to health care.

Clearly there are parallels between the developments in the health arena and developments in the larger society, some perhaps circumstantial and other less so. Just as the economic sector suffered at the point of production from insufficient decentralization, so the health system suffered at the point of primary services from insufficient focus of resources in the polyclinic. Just as the large-scale mobilization approach in the economy created insufficient clarity of responsibility and accountability, so the assignment of physicians for certain hours or days to the polyclinic failed to sustain either the teamwork or the individualized accountability required for patient and community health affairs.

The conditions which pressed upon the society for criticism and experimentation in 1970 similarly affected the health system. The Plaza experiment emerged in the initial period of post-1970 debate. The Alamar project coincided with the Matanzas experiment, and in Matanzas province itself, the Reynol García model polyclinic was promptly established. I was hopeful that in Matanzas I would be able to see what might be some of the effects on the health system of the new sociopolitical organization. It was, however, too early to see, and health services appeared directed through the usual lines of the ministry, and not from the local government. The character of the health commissions was being influenced by the participation by municipal assembly delegates, and the assembly was setting up its own health commission. Local health matters were expected to fall more closely under local direction when the boundaries designated by the new constitution were effected, as they were, later in 1976. Matanzas province became two — Matanzas and Gerón. Meanwhile, the voices of medicine in the community have heralded the moves toward decentralization and democratization as certain, or at least prerequisite, to the full development of lay leadership in health. Personally, I am convinced that this will be the case; for the new measures will introduce stability in lay influence, and the weight of a local institution such as the municipal peoples' assembly will press heavily against the previous orientation of thinking in terms of multiple national-local hierarchies of authority.

OTHER DEVELOPMENTS IN HEALTH CARE

Medical training of all kinds has constantly undergone decentralization. Almost all nonphysician training programs, including nursing, are found complete in the seven health provinces. Even medical students are now spending their clinical years of training (third through sixth) in provincial teaching centers. Only the first two years of preclinical studies are necessarily spent in Santiago, Santa Clara, or Havana.

Cuba appears to be succeeding in lowering the infant and maternal mortality rates, in accord with goals set in 1970. When, in 1969, the trend of decreasing infant mortality reversed itself and registered a small but definite increase to 48.9 per 1,000 live births, an intense campaign was launched, setting as its goal the reduction of the rate to 20.0, precisely, by coincidence, the 1970 rate for the United States. At the same time, maternal mortality (8.8 per 10,000 live births in 1969) was to be lowered to 2.0 (compared to the 1970 rate in the United States of 2.2). Studies of regional distributions of mortality and resources were conducted, aimed at focusing programs in the areas of greatest severity. Maternal education emphasized prenatal attention, breast feeding, and general nutrition. In rural areas, a new kind of institution, the nutritional recovery home, similar to the maternal homes for prebirth stays, was created. Here, high-risk children are placed after release from hospitalization, promoting maternal living-in and aiming the experience toward health education. By 1973, the infant mortality had fallen to 27.4 per 1,000 live births and the maternal mortality rate had declined to 5.2 per 10,000 live births.[16]

Hospital development continues, and the first major hospital facility to have been built in Havana by the revolutionary government is now receiving some of the scientific institutes which had been located in antiquated facilities. The new building towers thoughtfully over the ruins of the old poorhouse, the Casa de Beneficencia, to which Tomás Romay had sung praises in 1799. Part of the ruins are apparently being preserved, at least the *turno*, a half-sized doorway where, until 1963, parents were provided a sanctioned and anonymous means for abandoning their infants, dropping them at nighttime through the swinging door. (A bell, which rang when the baby fell through the door, alerted the waiting sisters of charity.) In other areas, hospital investment appears to be mostly guided by the goals of maternal-infant care.

Three new scientific institutes are in process of development: nutrition, occupational medicine, and health development. The Institute for Health Development is moving into the old Lebredo tuberculosis hospital (reflecting a change in that treatment mode), which was renovated by the Ministry's mini-brigades. This institute is primarily concerned with issues of health administration, planning, and statistics, topics which now find expression in the institute's journal, the *Revista Cubana de Administración de Salud*. A closely associated Cuban Society of Health Administration was formed in 1974, with membership sections on medicine in the community, medical education, planning, and biostatistics and demography. This society is already influential, contributing to the institute and its journal and lending support to administrative innovation and implementation of medicine in the community. The creation of the new institutes is yet another step in determining a balance of social and clinical medicine.

DENTISTRY-ESTOMATOLOGY

Among the serious shortcomings, thusfar, of my analysis of Cuban health care, one of the most painful is the scant reference to dentistry. By juxtaposing dentistry to the rest of medicine, the notable features of both will stand out.

While dental education was brought into the University of Havana in the course of the first North American intervention, dentistry maintained its professional organization and its school separate from the rest of medicine. In some respects, the professional association of dentists (the Colegio Dental) was more powerful than the medical profession. Unlike the medical school, the dental school managed to sharply limit the number of students, notwithstanding many students strikes and demonstrations in opposition to this measure. Thus, without a "plethora" of dentists, but with a problem of dental emigration, the contemporary revolutionary period began with a very severe shortage of dentists. This shortage has never been wholly corrected, and every plan since 1963 speaks of this issue. The unification of dentistry and medicine, giving dentistry the name of estomatology, did not serve to introduce large numbers of new students into dentistry, but their preparation was improved.

On first glance, then, dentistry is integrated into medicine, with posts specified in plans for polyclinics and regional hospital facilities. In truth, however, the physical presence of estomatologists in the polyclinic is not universal, and depends on the relationship of the polyclinic to other available dental services that evolved in the process of rationalizing dentistry and making maximum use of scarce resources. The special services of dentistry that grew in this process were found in *dental clinics*, particularly in urban areas. Actually, all of the polyclinics that I visited in Cuba in 1968 and in 1976 offered the services of an estomatologist, but they referred much of their dental work to clinics, when they were accessible. This was true in Havana, Cienfuegos, and Camagüey.

Dentistry, by offering free services, experienced, like medicine generally, a large demand for services but with greater resources limitations and the clear impossibility of soon overcoming such limitations by training more dentists. But as many dentists emigrated, those who took authority for dentistry confiscated the abandoned office equipment (dentistry, unlike medicine, was primarily solo-office practice) and combined them in clinics where dental auxiliaries were rapidly trained and trusted in their use, employing some three dental auxiliaries for every dentist. Meanwhile, this development occurred simultaneously with another which greatly facilitated and even pressured for clinic, assembly-line procedures. The high-speed drill was developed at this time and it was imported to Cuba as part of the medical ransom that the United States paid for the return of the mercenaries captured at the Bay of Pigs. Thus armed with early experience and compatible new technology, clinic development progressed and was remarkably effective in meeting demands for services. In 1967, the training of dental auxiliaries was further formalized.

One dimension of clinic development is noteworthy. Owing to the priority of serving children and the difficulty of freeing working parents to bring their children to clinics, dental clinics were set up on a regionalized basis in the schools themselves. Thus, during the school day, students would receive dental examinations and treatment, including fluoride applications. There was, I think, roughly one clinic for every five primary schools in Havana in 1976.

Recently the use of auxiliary personnel, both assistants and auxiliaries (the latter are more highly trained), is being again transformed as estomatologists experiment with a variant of the New Zealand "four handed" approach.

Thus, while estomatologists (who have identical career and salary structures as other physicians) are increasingly pressured to think of themselves as physicians, they have a distinctive history both in the socialist and in the presocialist years. Their work has been highly innovative and is even considered by some to be more "revolutionary" than the work styles of other physicians. This is indeed interesting. Dentistry was a more conservative presocialist profession, but one consequence of its conservatism under the revolution was that it had to be more innovative in the use of personnel. Today, perhaps, the horizontal team collaboration between physicians and nurses will be comparable to the roles developed in estomatology.

NOTES

1. I suggest the use of the concepts, "organizational focus" and "focal organization" as comparative characteristics of national health systems in my "The Cuban Polyclinic: Organizational Focus in an Emerging System," *Inquiry*, special issue on comparative analysis of health systems, edited by Ray H. Elling, 12 (July 1975 supplement): 86-102.

2. Joseph Kahl, "The Moral Economy of the Revolution," in Irving Louis Horowitz, ed., *Cuban Communism* (New Brunswick, N.J.: Transaction, 1970), pp. 95-115.

3. Fidel Castro, speech of July 26, 1970, *Granma Weekly Review*, August 2, 1970.

4. A.R.M. Ritter, *The Economic Development of Revolutionary Cuba: Strategy and Performance* (New York: Praeger, 1974).

5. An excellent descriptive discussion of economic planning in Cuba is Armando López Coll and Armando Santiago, "Notas sobre el proceso de planificación en Cuba," *Economía y Desarrollo* 5 (January-February 1975) 1: 5-25. Anticipating structural changes in Cuba, the authors cite (p. 24) Fidel Castro's July 26, 1974 address in Matanzas:

> We are not just dealing with the question of centralization and decentralization, and it is not only that what pertains to the municipality should belong to the municipality, and so forth up to the nation. This experiment implies a step of transcendental practical and theoretical importance for the Revolution: they are the steps which should guide us toward the definitive institutionalization of the Cuban socialist State.
>
> The Revolutionary Government is a government of a provisional nature . . . but this provisional character has continued for more than fifteen years. It is necessary now to be thinking about the definitive form that the Cuban socialist State may take. And of course, that State must be constructed upon strictly democratic foundations.

6. D. Booth, "Cuba, Color and the Revolution," *Science and Society* 40 (1976): 129-72. See also A. Hagerman, "Women," in K. Ward, ed., *Cuba: People and Questions* (New York: Friendship Press, 1975).

7. Carlos Rafael Rodríguez, perhaps Cuba's most politically influential economist, blames the early undervaluation of the role of expertise on a kind of "radicalism from above" and not on worker resistance to technical direction. See Carlos Rafael Rodríguez, "En el proceso de construcción del socialismo la política debe tener prioridad," *Economía y Desarrollo*, 4 (1974): 155. This article is an extremely valuable interview by Marta Harnecker, director of *Chile Hoy*, first published in Chile in August 1972. The interview treats various themes of special interest to socialist theoreticians, particularly the elements of economic policy from 1960 to 1972.

8. Cuba, Ministerio de Salud Pública, *Anuario estadístico* (Havana: Instituto Cubano del Libro, 1975). Also, see Cuba, Ministerio de Salud Pública, *Organización de los servicios y nivel de salud, 1974* (Havana: Ministerio de Salud Pública, 1974). One may presume that the Cuban health statistics are good, because they believe in the value of statistics and use them as a guide to health planning. The statistics, as their collection improved, also show increases in morbidity and mortality categories as well as decreases. Statistical procedures were revamped by 1963 and were last revised in 1968. After at least 1968, Cuban health statistics have been considered the most complete in Latin America.

9. Cuba, Ministerio de Salud Pública, Dirección Provincial Habana, "Estudio estructural y funcional de los policlínicos de La Habana Metropolitana," mimeographed, no data of publication, 1974(?).

10. José A. Fernández Sacasas and Julio López Benítez, "El profesor en la comunidad," *Revista Cubana de Administración de Salud*, 2 (January-March 1976) 1: 1.

11. Ibid., p. 3.

12. Guillermo Barrientos Llano, "El equipo de salud en el primer nivel de atención," *Revista Cubana de Administración de Salud*, 2 (January-March 1976) 1: 12.

13. Ibid., p. 15.

14. Fernández Sacasas and López Benítez, p. 4.

15. Barrientos Llano, p. 19.

16. These and related statistics may be found in Panamerican Health Organization, *Health Conditions in the Americas, 1969-1972*, Scientific Publication No. 287 (Washington, D.C.: Pan American Health Organization, 1974). For statistics and discussion see: Cuba, Ministerio de Salud Pública, *Cuba: Organización de los servicios y nivel de salud*, pp. 73-88.

9
Review

This section does not close the history of health organization in Cuba nor complete its description. I hope that my work may have helped to open this aspect of the Cuban experience to English-language readers. Cuba's history provides rich material relevant to specialized interests, in particular, medical professionalism, the role of private social security, prepaid group practice, structural dynamics of health organizations, and the contribution of socialism to health care. Much remains to unearth from the past, to describe in the present, and to anticipate in the future. Specialized histories would greatly improve the grasp on history contained in these pages, notably on ethnic associations, mutualism, and government services in health and social security. A history of the health system in a single region or municipality would be a major contribution, and the visibility of the present system would be vastly improved by a careful descriptive study of an existing province of Cuba and of one region, municipality, and area within it.[1] The historical and present role of race and sex must be elaborated, and someone *must* attempt a history (or film or novel) of Enriqueta Faber. Descriptions of contemporary Cuban care of the aged, chronically ill, and the psychologically impaired are needed. Finally, we may look forward to examine the outcome of medicine in the community, the impact on health organization of decentralized government under the new socialist state, as well as the course of Cuban activities to improve nutrition, curb cancer, defend the environment, reduce automobile accidents, and level the professions. How does the health sector relate to homosexuality, abortion, alcoholism, and suicide?[2] It is essential that the social history of dentistry be examined in detail.

213

ADEQUACY OF THE HEALTH SYSTEM

My concluding objective is to analyze in a few pages the broad contours of the history that has been traversed in the preceding pages. Brevity, I hope, will allow the whole of history to come briefly into view and also avoid the inevitable redundancy of a really complete and detailed summary. A short examination of the adequacy of the changing health system will be followed by a review of the technological and structural dynamics of medical revolution.

Access to Official Care

A number of approaches might be useful to achieve an overall perspective. One such view would examine the differential accessibility of official quality care to the various sectors of the Cuban population. This view of system "adequacy" (as defined in part I, Concepts of Health Organization) would reveal a development from a very small overall availability to a large availability with decreasing variation by social class or by region. This development is made more important by the fact that, in early Cuba, access to the services of official versus unofficial quality health care made little or no practical difference, whereas in recent times, following a trend that began in the first medical revolution and was definitively set by the second, the difference between official and unofficial medicine and hygiene acquired enormous practical dimensions. In relative terms, that is, in relation to a retrospective evaluation of the importance of access to official medicine, one might reasonably conclude that the immediately prerevolutionary system of personal services was rather more inadequate than in 1610 when Licenciate Juan Tejeda served the population of Havana and *curandera* Mariana de Nava attended the population of Santiago de Cuba.

The first profound effect of the socialist period was to improve the distribution of physicians and other personal services among the rural and undoctored areas, and, excepting certain discontinuities during the period of transition, the consolidation of the area polyclinic has greatly improved the availability of services to the entire population. Significantly, one of the criticisms of the transitional period of the socialist period has been that the quality of medical services has declined. In the terms of this study, it may be suggested that quality of some services was sacrificed in the pursuit of higher quality for others and in the pursuit of adequacy of the whole system. From a point of view that extends beyond the acute stage of transition, it seems assured that services have also improved with respect to the dimension of quality. The conclusion, here offered, is that the several rationalizing trends in medical training, paramedical integration, and regionalization signal a great improvement that could not have been expected from the prerevolutionary system. This conclusion is offered, first, with respect to the clinical and technical dimensions of care and, second, with the human dimension. The humanization of care is improved by medicine in the community.

Considering the adequacy of hospital services, the system has ranged from relative adequacy in the earliest period, to extreme degrees of inadequacy and varying maldistributions in the nineteenth century and presocialist republican periods, to greatly improved adequacy under socialism. Hospital concentration, first in urban Cuba and second in mutualism, determined that services were *more* than adequate for one-tenth of Cuba's population and less than adequate for roughly half of the population. (Roughly the same may be said of physician services; and less extreme numbers would hold for sanitray services.) In early Cuba, the expected simple functions of the hospital could be served by a few permanent institutions and by improvisation against sporadic changes in health conditions. But in the one hundred fifty years before 1900, the magnitude of epidemic and the number of homeless and away-from-home (soldiers, slaves, sailors, and merchants) often reached proportions that seriously overburdened the capacity of simple, although always growing, institutions and varied improvisation.

In that period of some 150 years, yellow fever was the strongest factor in hospital development, while toward the end of the period, approaching 1900, medical technological developments made the hospital a preferred site for a variety of old medical services and a number of newly created services. Owing to the concentration of institutions serving the immigrant populations in the metropolis, the twentieth century began with a concentration of services in Havana. This concentration, and *overall* system inadequacy, in 1958, was probably even greater than under the height of Spanish rule in the 1860s and 1880s, when physicians, a variety of allied legitimate healers, and a few hospitals were scattered about the island, near population centers and sugar mills. These services were severely reduced, however, as physicians abandoned rural Cuba in the wake of two periods of devastating war at the end of the nineteenth century. As rural sanitary conditions worsened, urban sanitary conditions improved; as rural medical needs increased, services of real quality, many increasingly dependent upon a hospital or other institutional setting, were more than ever concentrated in Havana.

Resources for Health Care

By referring above to system adequacy, I am implicitly making assumptions about the history of resource availability, which is therefore important to review. The earliest inadequacy of official services was mitigated by a frail economy, while in the first revolutionary period the increasing availability of resources was a consequence of the prosperity of sugar, slaves, and coffee; of the semigovernment budgetary functions of the Sociedad Patriótica; of irregular efforts of Spanish administration; and of the mechanisms of religious and upper-class charity. The reorganization of the budgetary function, and economic recovery under direct U.S. intervention and expanding investment gave substance to the second medical revolution, along with the related but independently strong economic base of Spanish mutualism. While the latter continued under conditions of stable expansion through a period of increased immigration and economic expansion in the 1920s, the budgetary functions of government fell into disarray in good times and approached collapse in bad. These conditions were very important in determining the fate of the third medical revolution, for its central period of development, from 1930 to 1940, was conditioned by great economic difficulties, while neither its beginning nor end points, from 1925 to 1929 and from 1941 to 1945, were so characterized. While the frustrations of the 1930s turned towards pragmatic individualism and hence social inaction, the government under economic recovery reinforced popular cynicism toward the potentials of reform through budgetary means alone.

The exceptions were few: slightly improved availability of public services for working women during pregnancy and for their children, and improved services and social security for victims of industrial accidents. Meanwhile, renewed expansion of mutualism and private practice occurred quite naturally, again eclipsing the prestige of public services and government direction of the health enterprise. As a consequence of the dominant financial role of mutualism, pseudomutualism, and individual entrepreneurialism, a severe maldistribution of facilities and personnel became the natural Cuban condition. Mutualism and pseudomutualism created an abundance of marginal positions which not only exacerbated the problems of urban concentration but also institutionalized the exploitation of the physician by the physician. By contrast, the socialist medical revolution occurs under a reformed and greatly expanded government budget, as is demonstrated by the increase in the budget of public health services from $22,670,900 in 1958 to $180,241,300 in 1968.[3] (Although the 1968 figure includes mutualism, the 1958 figure does not.) With some increase in economic constraints, beginning in 1968, and again after 1974, the Ministry of Public Health has enjoyed considerable budgetary freedom and continues to plan for greater expansion in the years ahead. Indeed, it is now possible to ask whether the system is more than adequate (either more than the society can afford or needs, relative to other investments) a question which is bound to appear in the present period, characterized by increasingly integrated planning for health and economic development. In fact, the proponents for medicine in the community have said, in essence, that hospital resources (but not services) are more than adequate, causing personal and preventive services in the community to remain less than adequate.

MEDICAL REVOLUTIONS

For two centuries before Romay the technical productive forces in the Cuban health system were stagnant. The state of applicable health knowledge was ineffective, fragmented, and essentially unchanging. Health and illness were seen as composed of few ingredients, not altogether subject to rational or empirical analysis, and treatment involved numerous medicines and procedures but only a handful of real alternatives which were not subjected to scientific, empirical evaluation. The constant condition of resource scarcity — as in the case of the most highly ranked practitioners — was made less significant by the simplicity, lack of development, and ineffectiveness of the resources themselves. The chronic instability of health conditions, which was gradually increasing in scale (population size, concentration, and frequency of disease), was the only dynamic productive force. It produced only minor antagonisms with the static technical forces of production. Rendered problematic by the homeless and away-from-home, the extreme instability of health conditions implied the need for certain organized arrangements for health support,[4] whereas the state of health knowledge implied none. This, however, was a friendly contradiction. The already routinized technology of the practitioner could be rather easily implemented under conditions of increased scale. By the same logic, the system tolerated wide fluctuations of resource scarcity and improvisation in organized care. (This was less true, of course, for nontechnical resources such as food, kindness, and comfort.)[5]

The essential characteristic of the relations of production in health care was the formal, but ineffective, hegemony of the physician over a variety of other healers. Economic and social conditions of formal education and the virtual absence of such institutions, for most of the early period, inhibited the preparation of many physicians. The few that did exist, inadequately demonstrated the superiority of the physician's art, and so failed to stimulate effective demand for his services in a poor, highly stratified society. Such a setting mitigated the potential antagonism between the formal power of physicians and the flimsy occupational rights of the alternate healers, since their services were directed, although not exclusively, toward different sectors of the population.

The consumer of health services, and even in large degree the physician also, had no tools to evaluate the real curative powers of different practitioners, except in the roughest fashion and usually by reference to extraneous characteristics. Therefore, every practitioner was encouraged to cultivate a variety of irrelevancies to enhance his prestige: the severe clinical stare, intimidating costume, unintelligible remedies, and plain deception.[6] Hospital care, by contrast, could at least be evaluated for its piety, charity, comfort and graciousness; but this evaluation would not reflect on medical practitioners. In any case, the channels for frequent complaints were very indirect between patients and accountable officials.[7] The professions were internally unorganized because they had little need for one another in the everyday practice of their arts, with the notable exception of various arrangements between pharmacists and other practitioners. This disorganization contributed to the absence, in this prescientific period, of any organized research or evaluation that could produce effective new knowledge or its effective propagation.

The resulting ideological superstructure of the health system manifested itself in the authoritarian, elitist, and individualistic style of all practitioners, their careful mix of charitable and curative intentions, and claims to monopoly privilege over health care as a marketplace commodity. They were authoritarian because their arts, like those of priest or diviner, required arbitrary defense against challenge; elitist because each sought monopoly privileges, catering especially to wealthier patients. Charity, of course, defended everyone from charges of illicit wealth and privilege. This cluster of notions was consistent with the prevailing social structures and values, the pervasive preoccupation with illness, and the weak intellectual basis of the practitioners' arts.

Although in many ways the health system was internally disorganized, with room for conflict among lower practitioners, the cluster of productive forces, social relations, and ideology together constituted an internally consistent system of health promotion in early Cuba, unthreatened by external forces. We learn that in a sense, ignorance is bliss; a stable system of available services was created. The confident practitioners always knew what to do with their simple tools. From a sociological viewpoint, it is of less interest that many activites of health support hurt more than helped; the organization of a system is shaped by its technology even when it is ineffective.

The First Medical Revolution

Stability based on ineffective technology is vulnerable whenever effective new knowledge appears, and is the more precarious when authority within a system is derived from external, traditional hierarchies surrounded by transforming economies and social class. The Cuban health system, which crawled its way to the end of the eighteenth century, was artificially protected from mounting scientific developments by Spanish isolation. Financial and cultural dependency of the university and Protomedicato on metropolitan authority isolated these structures from nearby forces of change. At the same time, the diverted priorties and frail economic means of the king caused the institutions of medical education and governance, which were formally separate, to be weak and unexpansive in their security.

The forces of change presented themselves more irresistably in the last half of the eighteenth century within the economic sphere. In an environment of an expansive world economy and loosening ties to Spain; enlightenment, reforms in governmental administration, greed, and economic expansion became mutually supportive. The consequent spiral of socioeconomic phenomena spawned economic, social and cultural institutions, the rise of a new social class, and reactive collaboration by the Spanish government. Such developments, strongly linked to an enthusiasm with science in other fields of application, argued independently for changes in the health system and supported pressures for change that were internal to the health system. Medical members of the new bourgeoisie, supported by its expansive institutions, embraced and promoted new ideas of medical analysis and health care, although, with the exception of smallpox vaccination, the new medical science had not yet taken a wholly convincing applied form. Nonetheless, an essential thrust of the new science was to reduce the obscure elitism of medicine[8] and to develop greater collective orientation and organization among practitioners. Eventually this tendency was manifested on the highest level in the movements toward the founding of the Cuban Academy of Medicine. Falling short of destroying by direct attack the organized elements of the old system, parallel institutions were created in medical education and public health. Some of the institutions were new in purpose and design, reflecting, in part, an increase in administrative effectiveness in the society as a whole.

Economic expansion based on slavery and more effective or enlightened government increased the volume of health needs and also available resources. The government recruited personnel by improving their training, offering scholarships, and soliciting immigrant professionals. The partially planned increase in population by immigration, new towns, rural development, and slavery, called attention to social aspects of changing health conditions.[9] But while yellow fever and other diseases were subjected to increasingly scientific analysis, the rising numbers of immigrants, slaves, and soldiers called for an expansion of early hospital development. Growing numbers of physicians and the first separately organized dentists were accompanied by more hospitals and asylums. For the first time, the hospital was offered, though not very convincingly, as a preferred place for treatment. This development reflected the more prominent role of the physician in the hospital and the use of the hospital as part of organized medical education.

Certain aspects of health promotion came to be viewed as human rights in addition to being obligations of public and private charity. Smallpox vaccination supported a preventive dimension in the intellectual superstructure and concrete organization of health care. The predominantly religious ideology of charity was reduced under the superimposition of a more comprehensive spirit of noblesse oblige, a sense of social mission for the performance of public good deeds. Such a spirit seems to have been at once the product of more highly integrated European states (under the late influence of cameralism and mercantilism) and of the self-conscious organization of entrepreneurial elites, such as the men who formed the Cuban *amigos del país*.

The members of the Sociedad Económica must be remembered as a truly remarkable group of talented, energetic men. Private opportunism aside, they evidenced an exceptional public spirit. Not until the socialist revolution did there again exist in Cuba such a remarkable confluence of organized class interest, power, ideology, and responsible public service. The essential feature of the next period, from 1825 to 1898, is the absence of these characteristics, the decline of public spirit and pragmatic dynamism of the Cuban oligarchy, which was incompletely superceded by a new Cuban nationalism. One cannot but wonder what might have been the future of the Cuban health system if political independence had been achieved in this early period. Perhaps the institution of national autonomy could have created, under the leadership of men like Romay, an enduring system of public health work that might have provided stable incentives for public-spirited practitioners. As it was, when the United States occupied Havana at the close of the nineteenth century, General Wood was to report that every house was contaminated with smallpox, a dismal end to a century that had begun with the energetic introduction of smallpox vaccination. Work by Cubans in public health dwindled to isolated efforts, reserving to Spanish officials the direction and organization of the rather limited public health development.

The broad forces of institutional inhibition undoubtedly contributed to the conservative directions within the medical academy that are revealed in Finlay's early battles, but this tendency was also influenced by the incompleteness of the first medical revolution itself. Failing to contribute dramatic new cures, smallpox vaccination notwithstanding, the main contribution of the first medical revolution was an intellectual orientation. But an intellectual orientation with inadequate substantive application is easily reduced to sophistry, dogma, and the simple creation of new oligarchs. The scientific approach in medicine had not yet gained power by its own strength alone; the scientific orientation in medicine was first bolstered by the strength of contributions elsewhere offered by science, by the happy coincidence of encyclopedism (where some physicians were really general scientists), and by the new classes that already benefited from scientific contributions. Romay's work, as perhaps the best example, was greatly weighted by his social class and bureaucratic power.

The extraneous support for weak technical productive forces in medicine lends a quality of superficiality to the new order of the first medical revolution. While the new appreciation of anatomy improved the academic and professional role of surgeons in particular, the broad majority of practitioners experienced few changes, with the creation of a chair and regulations for pharmacy not occurring until 1842. Jenner's triumph of empirical observation remained the unequaled practical consequence of scientific medicine before the epidemiological observations by Snow and others of cholera in the 1850s and, at about the same time, the multifaceted implications of Pasteur's bacteriological and immunological discoveries.

The Second Medical Revolution

A victory of science intrinsic to personal medical services was finally possible, though not concluded, with the practical generalization of asepsis and antiseptic methods, and further developments in microbiology and immunology from 1880 to 1900. These developments of scientific medicine, together with the discovery of the mosquito vector of yellow fever and malaria, provided the key analytical forces which drove the second medical revolution. Its background is set by the disease forces themselves, nineteenth century advances in sanitary science, continuing immigration, war, the United States military occupation, the ending of Spanish domination, and, perhaps, Cuban national independence.

The remarkable combination of these phenomena spelled sudden improvement, after such extreme decline, in health conditions and health services. The kinds of effective health needs and demands for services changed with similar velocity. In spite of lowered levels of disease and disability, the demand for new medical products, and greatly expanding immigration, caused the expansion of all services, especially the medical and hospital services of Spanish mutual aid associations.

An irony may be offered to explain this turn of history. Under Spanish rule, a locus of public spirit, intelligence, and leadership was generated under the umbrella of the Creole social institution, the Sociedad Económica de Amigos del País. Under Cuban misgovernment, a similar source of quasi-public initiative lay with the Spanish, now outside of government, and their regional centers which, as has been said, provided for various needs, including the medical needs, of their members. The essential ingredients common to both institutions, (The Sociedad Económica and the regional centers) seem to have been the organizational flexibility of nongovernment status and the stability of leadership provided by a direct link to an economically solid constituency. The Spanish, now out of office, needed more than even their ethnic associations to maintain their health, business connections, jobs, social affairs, and solidarity. These very same functions were performed by the Sociedad Económica for Cuban Creoles before independence.

Responding to the flare for hospital technologies, physicians were seized with the fear of losing their patients, either to the programs of the ethnic centers, or to physicians with appointments or privileges in the remarkably improved public hospitals. In defense, patients were hospitalized in the homes of physicians, a practice not uncommon in earlier times, and enterprising physicians launched agressive new hospital-like clinics. The hectic prosperity of the 1920s caused the proliferation of every type of practice, especially the formation of new mutualist plans for otherwise private clinics. As new specialities emerged in the United States and Europe, new "fathers" of Cuban medicine appeared, either with faculty appointment, private clinic, or both. A young capitalism thus emerged in medical care, with farsighted entrepreneurs taking possession of new technologies.

As a consequence, the great development of social medicine and the new concept of preventive medicine as a human right were greatly overshadowed by the gleaming success of clinical medicine and its entrepreneurial exploitation. The effective development of social medicine depended on political support and public administration, a weak quality of the ambivalent republic. Thus, the benefits of both social and clinical medicine predominated in Havana and large cities, serving especially the wealthy and moderately well-to-do, a pattern of dazzling neglect that characterized the Cuban nation until the revolution of 1959.

In a very real sense, the second medical revolution was the completion of the first. Scientific method, gaining superiority as an intellectual device in the first period, yielded convincing practical technology only in the second medical revolution. Even smallpox eradication, begun by Romay, was completed under the direction of U.S. military intervention. The fruitless claims of superiority of hospital over nonhospital care made by Romay became reality in the second period, and the frail sanitary organization by the Sociedad Patriótica was finally realized in Cuban form by Secretariat of Sanitation and Charities of the Republic. Interestingly, the second revolution was marked by the application of ideas and methods introduced in the first period and also by the improved organization of previously existing practices, such as smallpox vaccination.

The Third Medical Revolution, 1925–1945

The consolidation of the final prerevolutionary system was not without its ambiguities and conflicts. As the economy stumbled and collapsed after 1929, conflicts came to the surface: between small physician-controlled clinics and large mutualism, between physicians as wage earners and physicians as capitalist entrepreneurs, and among physicians, mutualism, public facilities, and government. As larger numbers of young physicians joined the profession (and conservative physicians lacked the power to limit the number of medical students), there was a tendency toward greater identification as health workers rather than as individual entrepreneurs, and toward increasing demands by physicians for improved public services and public employment. But these tendencies within the Cuban Medical Federation were forever compromised and frustrated by political realities. Achieving limited success, the profession became entrenched, so to speak, in its hard-won victories, without having overcome the basic contradictions within the structure of services themselves.

The organizational challenge posed by the possibilities of twentieth century sanitary and medical progress continued to be largely unmet, although not without effort, beyond major urban boundaries, either by government, mutualist, or private practice. Meanwhile, the provision of adequate, if inefficient, services through mutualist and private practice to roughly half of Havana's population set a tradition of relative quality[10] that contrasted sharply with the public services for the remaining half of Havana. The latter services contrasted in turn with the services for much of the remainder of Cuba's population in what was so often called the "interior." Throughout the whole of the prerevolutionary republic, scientific advances in curative and preventive medicine exacerbated the meaning of the rural-urban dichotomy spelled by the contrasting availability of hospital services.

The third revolution was primarily an organizational product of the scientific revolution in medicine and can be reasonably regarded as the industrial revolution of health care, especially of its hospital component. Its unique features, mutualist organization and a confused combination of employee-physicians and private practitioners, are probably best understood as an outgrowth of a unique feature of the previous revolutionary period: the birth of the hospital functions of the regional centers and of the limited, but always ambitious, government health sector. While the development of a rigid structure of professional work is, in part, a reaction to technical developments, it should not be overlooked that technical progress continued throughout the period before 1959 and created growing tensions within the productive organizations of medical care, between the rigid professional structure and the personnel, educational, and organizational directions pressured by the forces of technology. The latter, for example, rendered archaic by 1959 the tiny private hospitals and small mutualist clinics. The third revolution failed to assault the principal contradictions of the health system and hence led not toward the new directions — rationalized urban concentration and extension to rural areas of greatest need — but rather to a rigidification of aging urban structures whose pattern was already set in 1930.

Nonetheless, the stymied third medical revolution created ideas, creative minorities, and technical expertise that would be reawakened in 1959, in the persons of middle-aged medical generations of 1933 to 1940.

The Socialist Medical Revolution

In several ways the fourth, or socialist, medical revolution is a continuation of the third. Only in the socialist revolution has the central dilemma of the third revolutionary period been resolved; the "plethora" of variously employed and underemployed physicians in Havana. The recent change occurred, of course, because the Cuban Revolution made possible what was impossible in the hopelessly cynical and forever stymied prerevolutionary sociopolitical context, the expansion of rural services and the rationalization of urban facilities and fragmented public health programs. Only in the socialist period has the organization of hospitals, specialist, and paramedical services achieved a form that was earlier suggested by scientific requirements. To the extent that the socialist medical revolution has extended sanitary and preventive health measures to rural Cuba, it is the organizational complement of Carlos J. Finlay's personal struggles on behalf of social medicine and scientific hygiene. A similar observation would apply to the relation between the socialist medical revolution and the founding of tropical medicine and parasitology as new scientific areas in the early republic.

The Cuban Revolution of 1959 occurs at a time when social medical concerns were finding new substance for development. It was increasingly realized that the expansion of specialties, greater size, and division of labor had two very important consequences: organizational problems of complexity and the fragmentation of the patient. Medical sociology in the United States, social and preventive medicine in Britain, and family and community approaches to medical care have evolved. Similar medical trends promoted social medicine, family health, and medical psychology within the Cuban medical school after 1959. Cuban medical psychology, always soul-searching about its role and historical bias of individualist orientation, has begun collaboration with medical sociologists and others in order to move towards a sociological approach.[11]

The difference between Cuba and elsewhere, in the progress of social medicine, is that in Cuba the orientation of social medicine is not forced by textbooks, but is implicit in new structures of health practice, new career expectations of medical students, new constituencies, and a new socialist state. The change from the early transformation to the consolidation of the contemporary system is marked by the lessened role of social medicine as separate courses and disciplines in medical education and the shift to a role of backup support for all teaching and clinical departments. Moreover, hygiene and epidemiology has been elevated to the most prestigious postgraduate specialty and is exclusively limited to the top-ranking medical students, a condition which contrasts sharply with other societies.

In the course of the contemporary period, the morbidity and, in particular, the mortality structure began to closely approximate that of the developed nations. This was an escalated continuation of presocialist tendencies. (Life expectancy was rising at a rate of one year per year in the presocialist period; it rose at a rate of two years per year in the socialist period.)[12] The early extension of services to underdeveloped and underserved areas and populations of Cuba naturally led, as a second step, to pressure for more of the kind of services demanded by new patterns of disability and by new familiarity and expectations for health care — expectations and models which were set, in large degree, by the presocialist system. There was thus, in addition to the first development of the periphery, an increased growth in central hospital services, even to the point of asserting contrary claims for health expenditures. The combined tendency (within rationalization) toward larger size of facilities and the newness of their use and administration produced an abundance of organizational pathologies which were harmful to the humanistic objectives of patient service and destructive to the goals of service integration at the periphery. The focus on the periphery was politically defined in 1965-1968 in the form of the area polyclinic. This ideological commitment, growing out of the disruption of prerevolutionary patterns of primary care and early overuse of hospital services, served, finally, to create the basis for a constituency which would drive the movement for medicine in the community after 1971.

It is interesting to note that the pathologies derived from hospital and specialist domination are ones which are observed in developed capitalist societies such as the United States. But in the present period of medicine in the community, these pathologies are being confronted in ways that are wholly uncommon to capitalist societies, namely by means of effecting the hegemony of primary care interests in the health system and in the community, in alliance with a process of increasing political control over the health system by local democratic assemblies of government. Given the truly immense power of sophisticated, hospital-based clinical medicine, such a transformation (not yet, or perhaps ever, complete) seems to have been favored in Cuba only by virtue of the political base presented by the popular and deep-going revolution in the larger society. It had been possible in pre-socialist times, due to rather unique Cuban conditions, for a large part, perhaps even a majority, of the medical profession to be progressive and favoring social medical reform. But *never* could they have achieved sufficient power to endure the polarization of class interests against more powerful colleagues within the profession without the support and guidance of a strong, progressive (and probably necessarily socialist) government.

In the contemporary period which is drawing to a close as the provisional revolutionary structures are supplanted by the new socialist state, the key developments of the health system, the rural service and the area polyclinic, created new constituencies whose conditions of work led to ideological developments and social movements in the tradition of social medicine. These constituencies pressured, finally, within the emerging ideology and framework of the socialist state, for the implementation of medicine in the community, the hegemony at once of the area polyclinic and of the ideology of social medicine within the health system.

In the long and torturous route since the late nineteenth and early twentieth century divorce of social and biological medicine,[13] the conditions of medicine and health have changed enormously, as have the necessary conditions for their reunification. In Cuba, the conditions for reunification seem to be favored, not only by the broad health goals of the revolution and the rationalized network of health services, but especially in the work conditions of the area polyclinic where — in alliance with community constituencies — the social, environmental, and biological factors of health promotion are concretely integrated in a single Cuban medicine.

NOTES

1. Peter Orris's work begins this approach and a valuable detailed sketch of services in the Escambrey region of Las Villas province is found in Cuba, Ministerio de Salud Pública, *Cuba: Organización de los servicios y nivel de salud, 1974*, pp. 36-38. The predominantly (60 percent) rural population of 209,899 was served by eight areas, with the following set of services: one regional hospital, six polyclinics, two area hospitals, six rural hospitals, nine rural medical posts, one urban medical post, one maternal home, and twenty-eight pharmacies.

2. Some controversy emerged from the detention of homosexuals during the 1965 campaign against bureaucracy and "la dolce vita" in Havana. Sensitive Cubans regarded this as abusive and pressured the Ministry of the Interior to cease the practice. The official attitude was changed to regard homosexuality as a medical problem. Abortion, as well as birth control assistance, was made available early in the Revolution (illegal but thriving as an illicit business before 1959), but such services were neither promoted nor widely publicized. Despite its dynamic population, Cuba did not regard itself as having a population problem. The intensive study and program of improving obstetric and neonatal services in 1970 identified morbidity caused by self-induced abortion. The vigorous program of sex and maternal health education programs which consequently developed include complete explanation of birth control and abortion. Previously, in 1968, such educational efforts were directed to women after the birth of their fourth child. The suicide rate, always high in Cuba in comparison with other nations, has remained constant, but death from

self-inflicted injuries has climbed to rank as the seventh leading cause of death: 2.4 percent of all deaths, or a rate of 13.9 per 100,000 population in 1974, compared with 11.7 in the United States in 1972. See Panamerican Health Organization, pp. 103, 116; also Cuba, Ministerio de Salud Pública, *Cuba: Organización de los servicios y nivel de salud*, p. 71. A discussion of the suicide rate appears also in Arnaldo Tejeiro Fernández, "La serie cronológica," *Revista Cubana de Administración de Salud* 1 (January-June 1975) 1-2: 67-68.

3. Ministerio de Salud Pública, *Diez Años de Salud Pública*, pp. 193-205.

4. Of course the asylum, hospice, or hotel function is not a health factor that disappeared after the colonial period. The most recent form is the provision of health and hospital services to rural work brigades, scholarship students and child care centers (the latter under the joint supervision of the Ministry of Public Health and the Women's Federation). Three groups that are favored by the revolution, they are allocated privileged resources. In Camagüey, Summer 1969, one hospital bed per twenty youths was provided for the 40,000 youths of the voluntary force, "Columna Juventud Centenaria." See Orris, pp. 52-53. See also Marvin Leiner and Robert Ubell, "Day Care in Cuba: Children are the Revolution," *Saturday Review* (April 1, 1972): 54-58.

5. Similarly, the competing private clinics advertised "first class hospital services," increasingly a diversion from an assessment of true quality care. The influential role of the consumer, amid the egalitarian ideology of the present era, must bring qualities of kindness, food, and comfort to the foreground for consideration, if also the need for "hotel" services. The development of parental "sleep-in" facilities in pediatric hospitals is such a contemporary development. In place of Christian sermons: health education.

6. For example, the common practice, early established, was that the practitioner who recognized certain courses of illness would diagnose all conditions as being very severe. If indeed this was the case, the physician would recommend prayer and berate the patient for not calling him sooner. If the patient's condition was ambiguous, the physician would offer grudgingly to try his best. In case of a simple condition, the physician would promise the frightened patient a sure cure. It is not surprising (given the human physiology) that some physicians became highly respected for their healing arts. Always an overmedicated society, it would be interesting to know if placebo medicine finds a place in today's Cuban medicine.

7. Separated by a gulf of social status and bureaucratic distance. This dimension has evidently been reduced in later periods.

8. Certainly this was a dimension which did not disappear in the nineteenth century and is probably found in the continuation of certain professional postures in contemporary Cuban medical education. Progress, in this regard, is evidenced in the practical orientation of the curriculum, in the rural voluntary work of students and physicians alongside other health workers and auxiliaries, and in the growing emphasis on popular health education and demystification of medical roles.

9. By some coincidence, it was also the rural thrust of the socialist revolution which most strongly supported a social orientation of Cuban medicine.

10. In view of the point argued by some critics, that Cuba is over-investing in physicians, it occurs that the determination to greatly expand the number of physicians is partly influenced by a desire to *democratize* the prerevolutionary "plethora" of services for the privileged.

11. See Sally Guttmacher and Lourdes García, "Health and Social Science in Cuba," in Stan Ingman and Anthony Thomas, eds., *Topias and Utopias in Health*

(The Hague: Mouton, 1975).

12. Francisco Rojas Ochoa, "Tendencias demográficas recientes y perspectivas futuras de la población cubana," *Revista Cubana de Administración de Salud,* 1 (January-June 1975) 1-2: 12-23.

13. See George Rosen, "The History of Social Medicine," in Howard Freeman, Sol Levine, and Leo G. Reeder, eds., *Handbook of Medical Sociology* (second edition) (Englewood Cliffs, New Jersey: Prentice-Hall, 1972).

STATISTICAL APPENDIX

Sources of data which appear in the appendix are the following:

a) Cuba, Junta Central de Planificación. *Compendio estadístico de Cuba, 1967.*
b) Cuba, Ministerio de Salud Pública. *Cuba: Organización de los servicios y nivel de salud.*
c) Cuba, Ministerior de Salud Pública. *Informe anual, 1976.*
d) Cuba, Ministerio de Salud Pública. *Salud pública en cifras.*
e) Cuba, Ministerio de Salud Pública. *Salud pública en cifras. 1967*
f) Farnós Morejón, A. "Los niveles de mortalidad en Cuba durante el siglo XX." *Revista Cubana de Administración de Salud* 3(October-December 1977)4: 351-364.
g) Cuba, Ministerio de Salud Pública, Subsecretaria de Economía "Publicación No.1."
h) Dechamp, C., and M. P. Troncoso. *El problema médico y la asistencia mutualista en Cuba.*
i) Escobar, R. "Creced y multiplicaos?" *Cuba Internacional*, No. 103 (May 1978), 12-15.
j) Martí, A. "Una conquista: la salud." *Cuba Internacional* No. 103 (May 1978), 33-40.
k) Pan American Health Organization, *Health Conditions in the Americas, 1969-1972* (Scientific Publication No. 287). 1974.
l) Roemer, M. I. "Health Development and Political Policy: The Lesson of Cuba." *Journal of Health Politics, Policy and Law*, forthcoming.
m) Torras, J. "Los factores económicos en la crisis médica," *Economía y Desarrollo* 3(July-August, 1963)4: 7-33.

Citation of sources is here listed in the form, "chart: source, page."

A-1:i, 12
A-2:i, 14;j, 33
A-3:c, anexo, 17
A-4:k, 16
A-5:k, 15
A-6:k, 13
A-7:k, 20
A-8:8, 21
A-9:k, 23
A-10:k, 23;c, anexo, 19;e, 11
A-11:k, 27;c, anexo, 43
A-12:c, anexo, 26
A-13:k, 17;b, 71
A-14:c, anexo, 29
A-15:c, anexo, 45
A-16:k, 43;e, 18
A-17:k, 47;b, 96;c, anexo, 45
A-18:c, 41
A-19:k, 38;c, 44
A-20:c, anexo, 42
A-21:c, anexo, 77
A-22:c, anexo, 80
A-23:c, anexo, 83
A-24:c, anexo, 72, 81,
85;j, 36
A-25:c, anexo, 69;k, 68
A-26:k, 64-5;e, cuadro 33;m, 15;h, 28-9;a, 46;c, anexo, 57;c, 31;b, 35
A-27:h, 28-9;m, 15;g, 14
A-28:c, anexo, 59
A-29:b, 50;c, anexo, 68;k, 226;h, 28-9;m, 30;g, 14
A-30:h, 28-9;g, 2;a, 47;b, 35
A-31:a, 46
A-32:a, 46-7;c, 49
A-33:a, 46;c, 49;b, 35-35-8;d, 34
A-34:a, 46;c, anexo, 49, 80;b, 35-8
A-35:c, anexo, 65
A-36:c, anexo, 65
A-37:c, anexo, 61
A-38:c, anexo, 68
A-39:1, m, 17-8, 21;g, 42;a, 41;b, 35

In assessing total expenditures for health in 1955, I have used the ministry's 1958 ratio of total budget to beds to estimate the expenditure per bed ratio in the non-mutualist sectors not administered by the health ministry (A-39). In hazzarding an estimate of beds and *(Continued on page 241)*

A-1. Population of Cuba, 1775-1975

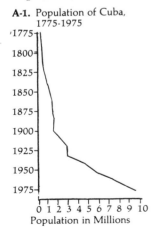

Population in Millions

A-2. Life Expectancy at Birth in Cuba, 1900-1972.

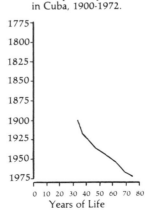

Years of Life

A-3. Deaths and Births in Cuba, 1800-1976. Rates per 1000 Population.

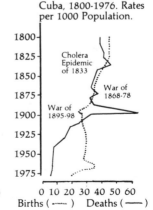

Births (·····)   Deaths (——)

A-4. Percentage of Deaths Due to Ill-Defined Causes in 14 Countries, 1972.

	0 10 20 30 40
Dominican R.	━━━━━━━━
El Salvador	━━━━━━━
Paraguay	━━━━━
Venezuela	━━━━
Guatemala	━━
Mexico	━
Colombia	━
Peru	━
Costa Rica	━
Argentina	─
Chile	─
Uruguay	─
United States	-
Cuba	.

A-7. Deaths from Infectious Diseases in 14 Countries, Rates per 100,000 Population, around 1972.

	Enteritis and Diarrheal Diseases	Other Infective & Parasitic Diseases
Argentina	23.9	42.6
Chile	35.9	45.5
Colombia	79.9	71.4
Costa Rica	54.1	46.6
Cuba	**9.7**	**17.8**
Dominican R.	60.9	38.9
El Salvador	117.9	58.2
Guatemala	265.8	288.4
Mexico	127.0	88.0
Paraguay	84.7	61.6
Peru	75.3	145.8
United States	1.2	6.6
Uruguay	10.7	21.7
Venezuela	51.7	47.6

A-5. Crude and Age-Adjusted Death Rates per 1,000 Population in 14 Countries.

	Period	Crude rate	Age-adjusted rate
Argentina	69-70	9.7	7.1
Chile	71-72	8.6	8.1
Colombia	68-69	8.0	8.3
Costa Rica	71-72	5.9	6.3
Cuba	71-72	**5.9**	**4.8**
Domin. R.	71-72	6.2	6.2
El Salvador	70-71	9.0	8.6
Guatemala	70-71	14.5	14.3
Mexico	71-72	9.0	8.4
Paraguay	71-72	9.6	9.7
Peru	69-70	8.1	7.9
U.S.	70-71	9.4	4.8
Uruguay	70-71	9.5	5.9
Venezuela	71-72	6.7	6.9

A-8. Deaths from Cancer of Trachea, Bronchus, and Lung by Sex (Age Adjusted Rates per 100,000 Population) in 14 Countries, 1971-72.

	Males	Females
	0 10 20 30	0 10
Argentina	━━━━━━━	─
U.S.	━━━━━━━	─
Uruguay	━━━━━	.
Cuba	━━━━━	─
Chile	━━━	.
Venezuela	━━	.
Paraguay	─	.
Costa Rica	─	.
Mexico	─	.
Colombia	─	.
Peru	─	.
Dom. R.	-	.
Guatemala	.	.
El Salvador	.	.

A-6. Life Expectancy at Birth in 12 Countries.

	Period	Life expectancy
Argentina	1970	65.7
Chile	1972	62.8
Colombia	1969	64.9
Costa Rica	1972	67.8
Cuba	1972	**71.2**
El Salvador	1971	65.0
Guatemala	1971	52.4
Mexico	1972	63.0
Peru	1970	65.7
United States	1971	71.4
Uruguay	1971	68.1
Venezuela	1972	66.4

A-9. Deaths from Heart Diseases in 1972 (Age Adj. Death Rates per 100,000) in 14 Countries.

	0 25 50 75 100 125 150
U.S.	━━━━━━━━━━━━
Argentina	━━━━━━━━━━
Uruguay	━━━━━━━━━━
Cuba	━━━━━━━━
Colombia	━━━━━━
Venezuela	━━━━━━
Chile	━━━━━
Costa Rica	━━━━━
Paraguay	━━━━
Mexico	━━━━
Peru	━━━
Dom. R.	━━━
Guatemala	━━
El Salvador	━━

A-10. Infant Deaths in Cuba and in Three Regions of the Americas, 1960-72 (Rates per 1000 Live Births)

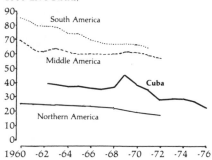

A-11. Maternal Deaths in Cuba and in Three Regions of the America, 1960-1976 (Rates per 10,000 Live Births)

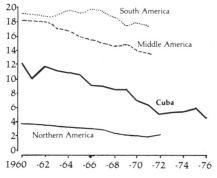

A-12. Late Fetal Deaths in Cuba, 1962-76. Rates per 1000 Live Births.

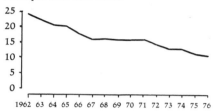

A-14. Ten Principal Causes of Death in Cuba, 1972-76, Rates per 100,000 Population.

	1972	1973	1974	1975	1976
Heart disease	135.4	144.6	155.8	148.3	156.8
Cancer	100.8	99.2	98.8	98.2	102.9
Cerebralvascular diseases	53.0	51.5	52.1	50.5	52.1
Influenza and Pneumonia	34.1	37.7	45.6	40.5	43.3
Accidents	31.8	31.7	31.4	32.7	32.4
Birth injury, dystocia, & other hypoxic conditions	36.9	32.6	28.7	25.2	20.1
Suicide and self-inflicted injuries	14.3	13.7	17.2	16.8	17.5
Congenital anomalies	14.1	13.3	12.5	11.8	10.9
Diabetes mellitus	10.0	10.0	8.6	9.1	9.9
Bronchitis, emphysema, and asthma	11.6	11.5	10.3	7.7	7.6

A-16. Reported Cases of Polio in Cuba and in Three Regions of the Americas, 1955-1973. Cases per 100,000 Population.

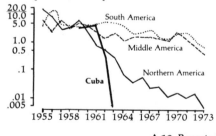

A-18. Deaths from Acute Diarrheal Diseases, in Cuba, 1962-76. Rates per 100,000.

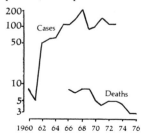

A-13. Five Principal Causes of Death in Three Regions of the Americas, 1970-72, and in Cuba, 1973, as Percentage of Total Deaths.

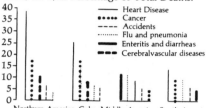

———— Heart Disease
••••• Cancer
– – – Accidents
·········· Flu and pneumonia
━━━ Enteritis and diarrheas
■■■ Cerebralvascular diseases

Northern America Cuba Middle America South America

A-15. Fourteen Diseases of Obligatory Notification in Cuba, 1965 and 1972-1976. Notified Cases per 100,000 Population.

	1965	1972	1973	1974	1975	1976
Typhoid fever	3.0	5.1	3.5	3.7	4.0	4.3
Tuberculosis	63.5	14.3	15.4	15.4	14.2	13.5
Tubercular meningitis	0.0	0.0	0.0	0.0	0.0	0.0
Leprosy	4.2	3.5	2.9	3.3	3.6	4.2
Dipheria	8.0	0.0	—	—	0.0	0.0
Whooping cough	26.6	14.3	23.8	18.0	3.5	1.5
Tetanus	6.5	1.7	1.1	1.0	0.7	0.6
Infantile tetanus	1.3	0.0	—	—	—	—
Measles	118.8	59.9	78.3	150.9	113.4	157.2
Human rabies	—	0.0	0.0	0.0	0.0	0.0
Malaria	1.6	0.4*	0.1*	0.4*	0.9*	1.9*
Meningocbal meningitis	0.3	0.5	0.3	0.4	0.3	0.8
Blenorrhea	8.9	7.9	9.6	35.2	47.0	65.8
Syphilis	29.7	24.3	48.9	50.5	47.6	41.1

*Imported cases.

A-17. Reported Cases of Tuberculosis per 100,000 Population in Cuba and Three Regions of the Americas, 1960-72.

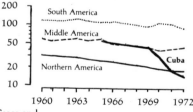

A-19. Reported Cases and Deaths from Infectious Hepatitis in Cuba, 1960-76. Rates per 100,000 Population.

A-20. Deaths from Motor Vehicle and Other Transport Accidents in Cuba, 1955-76. Rates per 100,000.

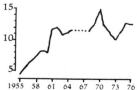

A-21. Medical and Dental Ambulatory Visits in Cuba, 1963-75. Visits per Habitant.

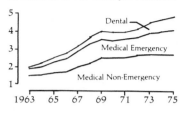

A-22. Ambulatory Visits per Habitant by Province, 1966 and 1975, Excluding Emergency Services.

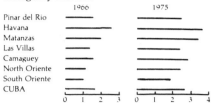

A-23. Percentage Distribution of Emergency and Non-Emergency Ambulatory Visits by Type of Facility, 1967 & 1975.

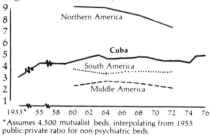

A-24. Maternal and Infant Non-Emergency Care. Proportion of Institutional Deliveries, Pre-Natal Visits, and Infant Visits per Live Birth, 1963-76.

	Inst. Births	Pre-Natal Visits	Infant Visits
1963	.63		
1964	.67		
1965	.73		
1966	.78	4.5	
1967	.78		
1968	.85		
1969	.89		
1970	.92		7.4
1971	.96	7.0	7.8
1972	.98		8.8
1973	.98		9.5
1974	.98		9.8
1975	.99	9.8	9.8
1976	.98	9.3	

A-25. Hospital Utilization in Cuba, 1965-75, With Comparisons for Two Other Countries in 1972.

	Hospitalizations per Habitant	Average Length of Stay	Percent Occupancy
1965	10.4	12.4	76.5
1967	11.3	11.7	75.9
1969	12.3	10.8	76.8
1971	12.9	9.2	73.8
1972			
Cuba	13.1	9.0	75.3
U.S.	15.7	8.5	75.9
Dom. R.	8.3	7.2	71.9
1973	13.2	9.0	76.9
1975	13.4	9.1	81.2

A-26. Hospital Beds per 1000 Population in Cuba, 1933, 1955, 1958-76, and in Three Regions of the Americas, 1960-72.

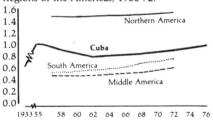

*Assumes 4,500 mutualist beds, interpolating from 1955 public:private ratio for non-psychiatric beds.

A-27. Physicians per 1000 Population in Cuba, 1933, 1955, 1958-76, and in Three Regions of the Americas, 1960-72.

A-28. Hospital Beds per 1000 Population and Relative Growth Factor, by Province, 1958-1976.

	1958	1976	Growth
Pinar del Rio	2.2	4.0	1.8
Havana	9.1	7.6	.84
Matanzas	2.3	4.6	2.0
Las Villas	2.6	3.7	1.4
Camaguey	2.7	5.3	2.0
Oriente	2.0	3.7	1.9
CUBA	4.2	5.0	1.2

A-29. Physicians per 1000 Inhabitants in Cuba, by Province, for Selected Years, 1933-1976.

	1933	1955	1958	1968	1972	1976
Pinar del Rio	0.38	0.47	0.46			
Havana	1.40	2.50	2.40		1.25	
Metro	2.20	3.10	4.00			
Non-Metro	0.49	0.63	0.63			
Matanzas	0.49	0.70	0.66			
Las Villas	0.39	0.60	0.59			
Camaguey	0.43	0.65	0.60			
Oriente	0.32	0.40	0.38			
CUBA	0.64	1.00	0.90	0.85	0.92	1.10

A-30. Comparison of Mutualist and Non-Mutualist Sectors in Cuba, 1933 and 1958.

	1933	1958
MUTUALISM*		
Beds per 1000 Members	14.4	10.0
Physicians per 1,000	2.4	2.0
NON-MUTUALISM		
Beds per 1000 People	2.1	3.1
Physicians per 1,000	0.49	0.74

*1933 estimates are very gross. I estimate 4,500 beds, 766 physicians, and 312,150 members in 1933 and 10,000, 2,000, and 1,000,000, respectively, in 1958.

A-33. Tuberculosis Hospitals in Cuba, Numbers and Beds, 1962-76.*

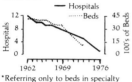

*Referring only to beds in specialty hospitals.

A-36. Graduation of Dentists, 1959-76.

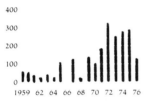

(Continued from page 237)

physicians in mutualism, I have assumed that (1) there was little change between 1958 and 1963; (2) that the number of physicians in mutualism equals the difference between 1962 and 1963 for physicians on the ministry payroll (as the mutualist payroll was integrated with the ministry) minus the number of medical graduates of the previous two years; (3) that the physician/bed ratio is the same in 1933 as in 1958. To estimate 1933 mutualist beds, I assumed that the ratio of ministry general beds to mutualist beds was constant in Havana. For beds of the interior, I chose the average of an estimate using the same method and my previous estimate (obviously an underestimate) obtained for Table 5.4. The number of mutualist members are taken for 1958 from the source cited, and for 1933 from Table 5.3 for Havana and from an assumption that the bed/member ratio of the interior was the same as Havana's.

A-31. Decline of Mutualist Beds, in Thousands, 1959-70.

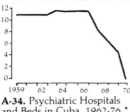

A-34. Psychiatric Hospitals and Beds in Cuba, 1962-76.*

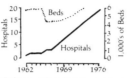

*Referring only to beds in specialty hospitals. There were 612 psychiatric beds in general hospitals in 1969

A-37. Graduates of Other Medical Training Programs, Totals for 1959-76.

General Nursing	7,833
Specialty Nursing	2,517
Nursing Aide	25,889
Dental Assistant	1,204
Pharmacy and Assistants	4,619
Sanitary Workers	2,015
Laboratory Technologist	4,993
X-Ray Technician and Aides	1,626
Others	10,928
Total	61,674

A-32. Polyclinics and Other Health Facilities 1962 & 1976.

	1962	1976
Polyclinics	161*	345
Rural Posts	52**	140
Dental Clinics	n. a.***	115
Public Health Laboratories	n. a.***	37
Blood Banks	2	21
Pediatric Recovery Homes	1	
Maternity Homes	n. a.***	62
Rural Hospitals	41****	57

*Includes 90 prerevolutionary municipal aid stations.
**Numbers for 1964.
***None in 1958.
****One in 1958.

A-35. Graduation of Physicians, 1959-76.

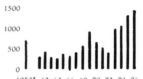

*Includes two classes.

A-38. The Labor Force in Cuban Health Care, 1976.

Physicians	9,985
Dentists	2,291
Pharmacists	658
Engineers	68
Other University Graduates	669
Nurses	9,710
Dental Assistants	1,045
Laboratory Technologists	4,139
X-Ray Technicians	1,150
Nursing Aides	13,787
Other Technicians	15,574
Skilled Workers	13,101
Unskilled Workers	9,778
Other Services & Administration	56,247
Total	138,201

A-39. National Resources Destined to Health Care, 1955 and 1976, in Millions of Pesos, Unadjusted for Inflation.

	1955		1976	
Payer	Pesos	(% National Income)	Pesos	(% National Account)*
Health Ministry	21	(1.1)	457	(10)
Other Non-Individual	13**	(0.7)	78	(1.7)
Individual	70***	(3.5)		
Totals	104	(5.2)	535	(11.7)

*Not having the figure for total National Account, I assume that the Ministry budget is still 10% of total government expenditures as it was in 1970.
**This is a maximum estimate, based on the number of beds in 1958 which were neither administered by MINSAP, or by mutualism.
***These 70 million may be thus distributed: mutualism, 27.6 (1.4); fee for service M.D.s, 12 (0.6); medicines, 21 (1.1); dentistry, 5.3 (0.3); hospitals, 1.9 (0.1).

Bibliography

Ackernecht, Erwin H. *History and Geography of the Most Important Diseases*. New York: Hafner, 1965.

Agrupación Católica Universitaria. "Encuesta de los trabajadores rurales, 1956-1957." *Economía y Desarrollo* 3 (July-August 1972) 12: 188-212.

"Alberto Recio y Forns (1885-1956)" (editorial obituary). *Revista KUBA de Medicina Tropical y de Parasitología* 12 (July-December 1956): 7-12, 47.

Amador García, Manuel, Physician of the Rural Dispensary of Bernardo, Baracoa, Oriente. "Enfermedad y condiciones de vida" (presented at the Tenth National Medical Congress, Havana, February 17-24, 1963). *Revista Cubana de Medicina* 2 (February 1963) 1: 34-45.

"Angel Arturo Aballí (1880-1952)" (editorial obituary). *Revista KUBA de Medicina Tropical y de Parasitología* 8 (October-November 1952): 10-12, 102-3.

Araujo Bernal, Leopoldo and Monteagudo, Gloria. "Experiencia derivada de una práctica social realizada por alumnos de medicina." *Revista Cubana de Medicina* 5 (December 1966) 6: 673-84.

Araujo Bernal, Leopoldo. "Psicología Social: Un enfoque sobre sus límites y conceptos básicos." *Revista Cubana de Medicina* 4 (April 1965) 2: 129-36.

Barrientos Llano, Guillermo. "El equipo de salud en el primer nivel de atención." *Revista Cubana de Administración de Salud* 2 (January-March 1976) 1: 12-23.

Beato Núñez, Virgilio. "Historia de la parasitología y de la medicina tropical en Cuba." *Revista KUBA de Medicina Tropical y de Parasitología* 4 (January 1948) 1: 10-21.

Black, W. M. *Report of Major W. M. Black, Corps of Engineers, U.S.A., Chief Engineer, Department of Cuba, for the Six Months Ending December 31,*

1900 (a part of the *Civil Report of Major General Leonard Wood on Cuba, 1900*). Washington, D.C.: U.S. Government Printing Office, n.d.

Boorstein, Edward. *The Economic Transformation of Cuba.* New York: Monthly Review Press, 1968.

Booth, D. "Cuba, Color and the Revolution." *Science and Society* 40 (1976): 129-72.

Bourne, Edward Gaylord. *Spain in America, 1450-1580* (first published, New York: Harpers, 1904). New York: Barnes and Noble, 1962.

Calvó Fonseca, Rafael, Finlay Institute. "Servicio de Salud en el medio rural: Proyecto de Organización Sanitaria-Asistencial." *Revista KUBA de Medicina Tropical y de Parasitología* 15 (January-June 1959) 1-6: 8-15.

Castro, Fidel. "On the Opening of the Polyclinic in Valle del Perú." *Granma* (English language edition, January 19, 1969): 1-3.

Castro, Fidel. Speech of July 26, 1970. *Granma Weekly Review* (August 2, 1970).

Colegio Médico de La Habana. *Relación de Médicos, 1945* (pamphlet, no facts of publication).

Commission on Cuban Affairs. *Problems of the New Cuba* (Wilson George Smillie, primary author of section on public health). New York: Foreign Policy Association, 1935.

Cuba. *Directorio Professional de Medicina y Farmacia de la República de Cuba.* Havana: Rambla, Bouya, 1929.

Cuba. Ministerio de Salud Pública. *Anuario estadístico.* Havana: Instituto Cubano del Libro, 1975.

Cuba. Ministerio de Salud Pública. *Diez años de salud pública.* Havana: Instituto del Libro, 1969.

Cuba. Ministerio de Salud Pública. *Organización de los servicios y nivel de salud, 1974.* Havana: Ministerio de Salud Pública, 1974(?).

Cuba. Ministerio de Salud Pública, Dirección Provincial Habana. "Estudio estructural y funcional de los policlínicos de La Habana Metropolitana." mimeographed, no data of publication, 1974(?).

Cuba. Ministerio de Salud Pública, Subsecretaria de Economía. *Publicación No. 1, Datos y cifras en salud pública, 1962* (pamphlet) Havana: Ministerio de Salud Pública, n.d.

Danielson, Ross. "The Cuban Polyclinic: Organizational Focus in an Emerging System." *Inquiry.* Special issue on comparative analysis of health systems, ed. Ray H. Elling. 12 (July 1975 supplement): 86-102.

de Arce, Louis A. "El Real Hospital Nuestra Señora del Pilar en el siglo XVIII (un hospital para los esclavos del Rey), 1764-1793." *Cuadernos de Historia de Salud Pública, no. 41.* Havana: Ministerio de Salud Pública, 1969.

Dechamp, Cyrille, and Moisés Poblete Troncoso. *El problema médico y la asistencia mutualista en Cuba* (a report of the International Labor Office). Havana, 1934.

de Geyndt, Willy. "The Cuban Hospital System." *World Hospitals* 8 (March 1970) 3: 280-86.

de Laura, María Julia. "Laura Martínez de Carvajal y del Camino (primera graduada de medicina en Cuba), en el septuagéximo quinto aniversario de su graduación (15 de julio de 1889)." *Cuadernos de Historia de la Salud Pública, no. 28.* Havana: Ministerio de Salud Pública, 1964.

del Pino y de la Vega, Mario, "Apuntes para la historia de los hospitales de Cuba (1523 a 1899)" *Cuadernos de Historia de Salud Pública, no. 24.* Havana: Ministerio de Salud Pública, 1963.

Dihigo, Mario E., "Recuerdos de una larga vida." *Cuadernos de Historia de la Salud Pública, no. 60.* Havana: Ministerio de Salud Pública, 1974.

"Dr. Carlos J. Finlay and the "Hall of Fame" of New York." *Booklet on Sanitation History, no. 15.* Havana: Ministry of Health and Hospital Assistance, 1959.

Elling, Ray H. "The Hospital's Changing Position in the Community," in Ray H. Elling, "Hospital and Community, A Study of Organizational Support" (draft of a book). University of Pittsburgh, 1965, chapter ii.

"El médico en las Instituciones Benéficas" (editorial). *Boletín del Colegio Médico de La Habana* 8 (March 1957) 3: 107.

"El X Congreso Médico-Estomatológico Nacional" (editorial). *Revista Cubana de Pediatría* 35 (February 1963) 6: 1-2.

Fernández-Conde, Agusto. *Biografía de la Federación Médica de Cuba.* Havana: Colegio Médico de La Habana, 1946.

Fernández Sacasas, José, and López Benítez, Julio, "El profesor en la comunidad." *Revista Cubana de Administración de Salud* 2 (January-March 1976) 1: 1-9.

Finlay, Carlos E. *Carlos Finlay and Yellow Fever.* New York: Oxford University Press, 1940.

Finlay, Carlos J. *Obras completas.* 3 vols., compiled with a biographical essay by César Rodríguez Expósito. Havana: Museo Histórico de Ciencias Médicas "Carlos J. Finlay," 1965-67.

Font Pupo, Carlos. "Hacia la salud pública socialista." *Cuba Socialista* 5 (July 1965) 47: 9-32.

Font Pupo, Carlos. "La salud del pueblo, preocupación básica del la Revolución." *Cuba Socialista* 3 (April 1963) 20: 41-60.

Font Pupo, Carlos. "Quinta reunión anual y extrordinaria del Cuerpo Médico del Centro Benéfico Jurídico de Trabajadores de Cuba, palabras del Dr. Carlos Font Pupo, Director de la Clínica, en la Aperatura del Acto." *Boletín del Colegio Médico de La Habana* 8 (April-May 1957) 4-5: 148-51.

"Forum Médico Nacional Sobre Seguridad Social-Mutualismo y Medicina Rural (octubre 30-31, noviembre 1ro, 1959." Havana: Archives of the Cuban Medical Federation, Museo de la Historia de la Ciencia "Carlos J. Finlay."

Freidson, Eliot. *Professional Dominance: The Social Structure of Medical Care.* New York: Atherton Press, 1970.

Friedson, Eliot. *Profession of Medicine: A Study of the Sociology of Applied Knowledge.* New York: Dodd, Mead, 1970.

Friedson, Eliot. "Review Essay: Health Factories, the New Industrial Sociology." *Social Problems* 14 (April 1967) 4: 493-501.

García Hernández, Manuel and Susana Martínez-Fortún y Foyo. "Apuntes históricos relativos a la farmacia en Cuba." *Cuadernos de Historia de Salud Pública, no. 33.* Havana: Ministerio de Salud Pública, 1967.

Gómez Luaces, Eduardo. "Regla: Su aporte a la medicina cubana en el siglo XIX." *Cuadernos de Historia de Salud Pública, no. 57.* Havana: Ministerio de Salud Pública, 1973.

Gómez Wangüemert, Luis. "Falsedad Desmentida." *Revista Cubana de Pediatría* 34 (September-October 1962) 5: 1-2.

González Prendes, Miguel A. "Informe del relator general." Presented at the National Conference on Norms of Leprosy Control, 1962. *Revista Cubana de Medicina* 1 (November-December 1962) 6: 45-50.

Guevara, Ernesto (Ché). "Visita del Comdte. Dr. Ernesto Guevara al Colegio Médico Nacional: Declaraciones del Dr. Guevara sobre la clase média." *Tribuna Médica* 20 (January-June 1959): 17-18.

Guttmacher, Sally and García, Lourdes. "Health and Social Science in Cuba." Included in Stan Ingman and Anthony Thomas, eds., *Topias and Utopias in Health* (proceedings of the Ninth International Congress of Anthropological and Ethnological Sciences, September 1973). The Hague: Mouton, 1975.

Hagerman, A., "Women." In K. Ward, ed., *Cuba: People and Questions.* New York: Friendship Press, 1975.

Hochschild, Arlie. "Student Power in Action." *Transaction* 6 (April 1969) 6: 16-21 and 62.

Ibañez Varona, René. "Historia de los hospitales y asilos de Puerto Príncipe o Camagüey (período colonial)." *Cuadernos de Historia Sanitaria, no. 6.* Havana: Ministerio de Salubridad y Asistencia Social, 1954.

Ibarra Pérez, Ramón and Sotolongo, Federico. "La Carrera Sanitaria." *Medicina de Hoy* 1 (September 1936): 3-5.

"José Antonio Presno" (editorial obituary). *Revista KUBA de Medicina Tropical y de Parasitología* 9 (July-December 1953) 7-12: 32.

Kahl, Joseph. "The Moral Economy of the Revolution." In Irving Louis Horowitz, ed., *Cuban Communism.* New Brunswick, N.J.: Transaction, 1970, pp. 95-115.

King, Lester S. *The Medical World of the Eighteenth Century.* Chicago: University of Chicago Press, 1958.

Knight, Franklin W. *Slave Society in Cuba During the Nineteenth Century.* Madison: University of Wisconsin Press, 1970.

Lage, Guillermo. "El primer hospital de la Habana." *Cuadernos de Historia Sanitaria, no. 3.* Havana: Ministerio de Salubridad y Asistencia Social, 1952.

Leiner, Marvin and Robert Ubell. "Day Care in Cuba: Children Are the Revolution." *Saturday Review*, April 1, 1972, 54-58.

Leland, R. G., Director, Bureau of Medical Economics, American Medical Association. "The Practice of Medicine in Cuba." *The American Medical Association Bulletin* 28 (June 1933) 6: 92-96.

Le Riverend, Julio. *Economic History of Cuba.* Translated by M. J. Cazabón and Homero León. Havana: Book Institute, 1967.

Le Roy y Gálvez, Luis Felipe. "Dr. Juan M. Sánchez de Bustamente y García del Barrio." *Cuadernos de Historia de Salud Pública, no. 42.* Havana: Ministerio de Salud Pública, 1969.

Le Roy y Gálvez, Luis Felipe. "Los orígenes de los estudios universitarios de las ciencias médicas en Cuba." *Revista "Finlay" de Historia Sanitaria* 7 (July-December 1966): 39-46.

López Coll, Armando and Santiago, Armando. "Notas sobre el processo de planificación en Cuba." *Economía y Desarrollo* 5 (January-February 1975) 1: 5-25.

López Sánchez, José. "Historia de la medicina en La Habana." *Cuadernos de Historia de Salud Pública, no. 47.* Havana: Ministerio de Salud Pública, 1967.

López Sánchez, José. "The Teaching of Medicine in Cuba: Its Past and Present State and Prospects of Its Future Development." *Revista "Finlay" de Historia Sanitaria* 6 (July-December 1965): 63-70.

López Sánchez, José. *Tomás Romay and the Origins of Science in Cuba.* Trans. Mary Todd Haessler. Havana: Book Institute, 1967.

López Serrano, Elena. "Apuntes para la historia: ingeniería sanitaria." *Revista Cubana de Administración de Salud* 2 (July-September 1976) 3: 307-19.

López Valdés, Jorge. "Organización de la asistencia psiquiátrica en el mutualismo." *Revista Cubana de Medicina* 5 (January-February 1966) 1: 62-81.

Martínez-Fortún y Foyo, José A. "Apuntes para la historia de la odontología en Cuba" *Cuadernos de Historia de Salud Pública, no. 23.* Havana: Ministerio de Salud Pública, 1963.

Martínez Junco, Heliodoro, et al. "Informe del Ministerio de Salud Pública a la Oficina Sanitaria Panamericana sobre el desarrollo del Plan de Salud durante el año 1962 y primer semestre de 1963." *Revista Cubana de Medicina* 3 (February 1964) 1: 6-22.

Mazorra, Oscar R. and Montero, Mario. "Estudio demográfico de 'Valle del Perú'." *Economía y Desarrollo* 3 (July-August 1972) 12: 188-212.

Mederos Torriente, Eleuterio, postgraduate in Rural Service. "El parasitismo intestinal en las montañas de Santa Catalina de Sagua de Tánamo." Presented at the Tenth National Medical Congress, Havana, February 17-24, 1963. *Revista Cubana de Medicina* 2 (February 1963) 1: 57-62.

Moll, Aristedes A. *Aesculapius in Latin America.* Philadelphia: W.B. Saunders, 1944.

Nájera, Luis. "Sobre la reforma de la enseñanza de la higiene y medicina preventiva en las facultivas de medicina." *Revista KUBA de Medicina Tropical y de Parasitología* 10 (July-December 1954) 7-12: 42-45.

Navarro, Vincente. "Health, Health Services, and Health Planning in Cuba." *International Journal of Health Services* 2 (August 1972) 3: 397-432.

Oficina Internacional del Trabajo. "Informe al Gobierno de Cuba sobre seguridad social." Geneva: International Labor Office, 1960, mimeographed.

Orris, Peter. "The Role of the Consumer in the Cuban Health System." Unpublished dissertation, master of public health. Yale University, 1970.

Panamerican Health Organization. *Health Conditions in the Americas, 1969-1972* (Scientific Publication No. 287). Washington, D.C.: Panamerican Health Organization, 1974.

Paulís Pagés, J. and Monteros-Valdivieso, M. Y. *Joaquín Albarrán: General artífice de la Urología.* Havana: Museo Histórico de las Ciencias Médicas "Carlos J. Finlay," 1963.

Perera, Ambrosio. *Historia de la medicina en Venezuela.* Caracas: Ministerio de Sanidad y Asistencia Social, Imprenta Nacional, 1951.

Pérez de la Riva, Juan. "Cuántos africanos fueron traídos a Cuba?" *Economía y Desarrollo* 1 (July-September 1970) 3: 139-43.

Perrow, Charles. "A Framework for the Comparative Analysis of Organizations." *American Sociological Review* 32 (April 1967) 2: 194-208.

Perrow, Charles. "Goals and Power Structures: A Historical Case Analysis." In Eliot Freidson, ed., *The Hospital in Modern Society.* Glencoe, Illinois: The Free Press, 1963, 112-46.

Perrow, Charles. "Hospitals: Technology, Structure, and Goals." In James March, ed., *Handbook of Organizations.* Chicago: Rand McNally, 1965.

Portuondo de Castro, Juan M. *Como se apoderaron los comunistas de la Universidad de La Habana.* Miami: Ediciones del Directorio Magisterial Cubano (Exilio), n.d.

Ritter, A.R.M., *The Economic Development of Revolutionary Cuba: Strategy and Performance,* New York: Praeger, 1974.

Rodríguez, Carlos Rafael. "En el proceso de construcción del socialismo la política debe tener prioridad." *Economía y Desarrollo* 4 (1974): 144-57.

Rodríguez Expósito, César. *Dr. Juan Guiteras.* Havana: Editorial Cubanicán, 1947.

Rodríguez Expósito, César. "Índice de médicos, dentistas, farmacéuticos y estudiantes en la guerra de los diez años. *Cuadernos de Historia de Salud Pública, no. 40.* Havana: Ministerio de Salud Pública, 1968.

Rodríguez Expósito, César. "La primera secretaria de sanidad del mundo se creó en Cuba. *Cuadernos de Historia de Salud Pública, no. 25.* Havana: Ministerio de Salud Pública, 1964.

Rodríguez Rivera, Luis. "Métodos de dirección colectiva en nuestra actual organización hospitalaria." *Revista Cubana de Medicina* 3 (August 1964) 4: 388-95.

Roemer, Milton I. "Medical Care and Social Class in Latin America." *Milbank Memorial Fund Quarterly* 42 (July 1964) 3, part I: 54-64.

Roemer, Milton I. *Medical Care in Latin America.* Washington, D.C.: General Secretariat, Organization of American States, 1963.

Roemer, Milton I. "World Trends in Medical Care Organization." *Social Research* 26 (Autumn 1959) 2: 283-310.

Roig de Leuchsenring, Emilio. *Médicos y medicina en Cuba: Historia, biografía, costumbrismo.* Havana: Museo Histórico de las Ciencias Médicas "Carlos J. Finlay," 1965.

Rojas Ochoa, Francisco, Director, Planning and Statistics Group, Ministry of

Public Health. "El policlínico y la asistencia a pacientes ambulatorios en Cuba." *Revista Cubana de Medicina* 10 (March-April 1971) 2: 214-15.

Rojas Ochoa, Francisco. "La red hospitalaria del Ministerio de Salud Pública en el período 1958-1969." *Revista Cubana de Medicina* 10 (January-February 1971) 1: 3-42.

Rojas Ochoa, Francisco. "Tendencias demográficas recientes y perspectivas futuras de la población cubana." *Revista Cubana de Administración de Salud* 1 (January-June 1975) 1-2: 11-16.

Romay y Chacón, Tomás. *Obras completas.* 2 vols., compiled with an introduction by José López Sánchez. Havana: Museo Histórico de las Ciencias Médicas "Carlos J. Finlay," 1965.

Rosen, George. *A History of Public Health.* New York: MD Publications, 1958.

Rosen, George. "The Evolution of Social Medicine." In Howard E. Freeman, Sol Levine, and Leo G. Reeder, eds., *Handbook of Medical Sociology* (second edition). Englewood Cliffs, New Jersey: Prentice-Hall, 1972, 39-60.

"Salus Populus" (editorial). *Boletín del Colegio Médico de La Habana* 8 (April-May 1957) 4-5: 145-46.

Santos Fernández, Juan. "*La vida rural.*" Speech before the Academy of Sciences, May 19, 1915. "*Cuadernos de Historia de Salud Pública, no. 16.* Havana: Ministerio de Salud Pública, 1965.

Santovenia, Emeterio S. "El protomédico de la Habana." *Cuadernos de Historia Sanitaria, no. 1.* Havana: Ministerio de Salubridad y Asistencia Social, 1952.

Segovia, Jorge and Omar J. Gómez. "Implicit vs. Explicit Goals: Medical Care in Argentina." Included in Stan Ingman and Anthony Thomas, eds., *Topias and Utopias in Health* (proceedings of the Ninth International Congress of Anthropological and Ethnological Sciences, September 1973). The Hague: Mouton, 1974.

Stich, Dr., Vice-Minister of Public Health of Czechoslavakia. "Coordinación e integración de los Servicios de Salubridad en Czechoslavakia." Presented at the Tenth National Medical Congress, Havana, February 17-24, 1963. *Revista Cubana de Medicina* 3 (June 1964) 3: 354-60.

Tejeiro Fernández, Arnaldo. "La serie cronológica" *Revista Cubana de Administración de Salud* 1 (January-June 1975) 1-2: 51-77.

Thomas, Hugh. *Cuba: The Pursuit of Freedom.* New York: Harper and Row, 1971.

Thorning, Joseph F. "Social Medicine in Cuba." *The Americas* 1 (April 1945) 4: 440-55.

Torras, Jacinto. "Los factores económicos en la crisis médica." *Economía y Desarrollo* 3 (July-August 1973) 4: 7-33.

Tressord, Manuel Michel and Robania, Orlando. Polyclinic of the Zone of San Luis. "Parasitismo intestinal en la zona rural." Presented at the Tenth National Medical Congress, Havana, February 17-24, 1963. *Revista Cubana de Medicina* 2 (February 1963) 1: 89-91.

Weinerman, E. Richard, with the assistance of Weinerman, Shirley B. *Social Medicine in Eastern Europe: The Organization of Health Services and the*

Education of Medical Personnel in Czechoslovakia, Hungary, and Poland. Cambridge, Massachusetts: Harvard University Press, 1969.

Wilensky, Harold. *Organizational Intelligence.* New York: Basic Books, 1969.

Williams, Eric. *Capitalism and Slavery.* New York: Russell and Russell, 1961.

Zeitlin, Maurice. "Cuba: Revolution without a blueprint." In Irving Louis Horowitz, ed., *Cuban Communism.* New Brunswick, N.J.: Transaction, 1970, pp. 81-92.

Index

Adequacy of health organizations: definition of, 9; in different historical periods, 214-17

Agrupación Católica Universitaria: and study of rural Cuba, 131

Alamar Polyclinic: as new model of health work, 198

Aldereguía, Gustavo: in prison under Machado, 104; and proposal for an alternative mutualist plan, 117

Area Polyclinic, 163; primary commitment to, 165; and hospital, 165, 168-69, 201, 206; teamwork in, 169, 200, 201, 203-5; growing utilization of, 170; and neighborhood sector, 171-72, 201; and health commission, 172-76; and rural health center, 177; and mutualism, 177-78; and *casas de socorro*, 179; and Czech Soviet models, 180; critique of by medicine in the community, 198-200; model of, given by medicine in the community, 201-7

Assessment Commission for Medicine in the Community: *see* Medicine in the community

Auxiliary personnel: training of, 183-84

Batista, Fulgencio: first appearance as strong man, 107

Blacks: and mutualism, 6, 120; and revolution in the medical school, 138; and the revolution, 192; *see also* Slaves

Borges, José Elias (physician martyr), 106

Bustamente, Juan M.: and medical education in nineteenth century, 71

Casa de Beneficencia: founded, 64; ruins of, 207

Centralization-decentralization: in the first socialist model, 145; in the prerevolutionary ministry, 145-46; effect of vertical task forces on, 148-50; and the area polyclinic, 165; of training of nurses and auxiliary personnel, 184; and the socialist constitution, 206; of physician training, 207

Centro Benéfico y Jurídico de los Trabajadores de Cuba, 120-21

Centros regionales: early development of, and yellow fever, 76-78, prominence of, 102; conflicts with the Cuban Medical Federation, 105-6, 107, 108, 115; *see also* Mutualism

Church: and folk healers, 22; and licensure, 24, 26; and charity, 27, 64; and monastic orders, 27; and slavery, 54-55; and smallpox vaccination, 54-55; and university,